T0073744

Patient-Centered Measurement

Patient-Centered Measurement

Ethics, Epistemology, and Dialogue in Contemporary Medicine

LEAH M. McCLIMANS

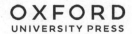

OXFORD
UNIVERSITY PRESS

OXFORD
UNIVERSITY PRESS

Oxford University Press is a department of the University of Oxford. It furthers
the University's objective of excellence in research, scholarship, and education
by publishing worldwide. Oxford is a registered trade mark of Oxford University
Press in the UK and certain other countries.

Published in the United States of America by Oxford University Press
198 Madison Avenue, New York, NY 10016, United States of America.

Library of Congress Cataloging-in-Publication Data
Names: McClimans, Leah, author.
Title: Patient-centered measurement : ethics, epistemology, and dialogue in
contemporary medicine / Leah M. McClimans.
Description: New York, NY : Oxford University Press, [2024] |
Includes bibliographical references and index.
Identifiers: LCCN 2023056800 (print) | LCCN 2023056801 (ebook) |
ISBN 9780197572078 (hardback) | ISBN 9780197572092 (epub)
Subjects: MESH: Health Care Evaluation Mechanisms | Patient Outcome Assessment |
Patient–Centered Care | Quality of Life | Hermeneutics
Classification: LCC RA425 (print) | LCC RA425 (ebook) | NLM W 84.41 |
DDC 362.1—dc23/eng/20240124
LC record available at https://lccn.loc.gov/2023056800
LC ebook record available at https://lccn.loc.gov/2023056801

DOI: 10.1093/oso/9780197572078.001.0001

Printed by Integrated Books International, United States of America

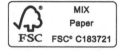

To the humans who helped me most: John and Georgia
To the animals who kept me together: Toni and Malcom

Contents

Contents

Acknowledgments

Writing this book has been a long journey. Like most journeys, there were many adventures along the way. My children were born, people I love died, I bought a horse, a pandemic came and went, I made countless journeys across the Atlantic, and all the while I was writing. It's not possible to continue a project like this one, with a life such as mine, without a lot of help. Sharon Reid and Sophia Reid-Recks looked after my children (and sometimes me) for years, giving us a sense of security and continuity that is rare. The kids hardly noticed when I was gone or working, for which I will always be grateful. My aunt Terri McClimans kept an eye on my mom when my mom was sick and I was in Ireland (or in a pandemic), taking a lot of the day-to day worry off my shoulders. Eimear White taught me how to ride my horse, remaining reassuringly stoic when I fell off, and generally provided me with a life-threatening distraction that made it possible to continue the work of this book. Ashley Duffalo, my oldest and best friend, took long phone calls from all over the world, listened carefully, and then gave succinct and practical advice. I wish I was more like you. Sally Williams has been listening and helping since the Royal College of Surgeons, when the ideas for this book were just barely beginning to take hold. *You are always on my side.* I am so lucky to have you. My colleagues at the University of South Carolina have been unfailingly supportive—of my research, of my transatlantic life, of everything. I am especially grateful for Chris Tollefsen, who has listened and advised me on innumerable life and work challenges with kindness and good humor, and sometimes food (but always wine); and Christine Caldwell, who has given me space on her futon, updates on pop culture, and a knowing smile.

Philosophy is such an unlikely way to earn a living. It's hard to explain to people outside the profession what you do; and frankly, sometimes it's hard to explain to yourself what you do. At the very beginning, Nancy Cartwright stood as an example of how to *be a philosopher*. Work hard, take it seriously, make a contribution, and don't waste (especially other people's) time. This mantra continues to play itself quietly in the background of my mind, and I'm so grateful to Nancy for it. It's been the philosophical making of me. But if Nancy made me want to make a contribution, it was meeting Eran Tal that helped me realize that aspiration. Sometimes you read or meet someone whose work speaks to you. Not just on the page, but what lies beyond the page. Such is the work of Eran Tal. And sometimes the author of that work is smart, humble, and generous. Such is Eran Tal. In philosophy, and I imagine other disciplines as well, there is an implicit expectation to "be smart," especially when asking questions. It is stressful. But I never feel like I have to be smart around Eran. It is *such* a gift for which I will always be grateful.

Long before Eran's work spoke to me, it was Gadamer's *Truth and Method*, and Georgia Warnke's work on Gadamer, that had me hooked. When the world is hard, when rejection seems to hover around the corner, when you aren't sure if you can make it, it's good to have someone who will hand you a glass of wine, listen sympathetically, and laugh at your stories. And if this person is also a first-rate philosopher who will read and comment on your work? Someone who lets you borrow the family pearls for your wedding and comes for the birth of your first child? Someone who hosts your three children and your babysitter for Easter? Even better. Georgia believed in this book—and me—before I did, before anyone did. Gratitude is too small a sentiment to accommodate this debt. Rather it is love. And respect. And admiration.

There are a number of philosophers, historians, and organizations that have shaped my thinking over the years and supported this project in big and small ways. Thank you to Anna Alexandrova for doing the heavy lifting of pioneering the work of integrating philosophy of science with well-being, and also for just being such a stalwart, intellectually generous, and kind person. Thank you to Becca Jackson for answering a lot of last-minute text message requests—philosophy emergency!—and for giving me hope that we have a new generation of History and Philosophy of Science scholars to wow us. Thank you to Sebastian Rodridguez Duque for reading drafts of this book and sending comments. You are a star. Thank you to Anderson Harris, who copyedited this book with such care and attention. Thank you to Sean Valles for writing interesting philosophy and giving advice via a last-minute Zoom call on how to get a book contract. Thank you to Hasok Chang, Rachel Ankeny, and Miriam Solomon for writing compelling philosophy (and history) that has served as an example of what is possible. Thank you to Suman Seth, who helped me with the title and read drafts, making this book *far* more readable than it was. You made me laugh and cringe and then laugh again (at myself). Thank you to Dan Hausman for always being interested and kind. Thank you to the Society for the Philosophy of Science in Practice for making me think for the first time that my work might have a philosophical audience. Thank you to the Society for the Study of Measurement, especially Luca Mari, for existing and giving us a place to showcase our work on measurement.

Part of taking my own philosophical work seriously has meant engaging with health researchers who work with patient-centered measures. While I started trying out my ideas on my husband (a health psychologist) as we planted vegetables in our London allotment, it soon became clear that I would need to go beyond the vegetable patch. He suggested I attend the International Society for Quality of Life Research's annual conference. I did, and it was just what I needed. I am so grateful for the support and kindness of this community, especially the members of the Response Shift Special Interest Group, in particular Caroline Schwartz, Bruce Rapkin, Nancy Mayo, Miriam Sprangers, and Jan Boehke. Philosophers of science who want to make a contribution to another field can't do so without the help and patience of those within it. Caroline, Bruce, Nancy, Miriam, and Jan, but also Joanne Greenhalgh, Stefan Cano, and Kevin Weinfurt, have suffered my questions and phone calls. Thank you so much. You have given me opportunities and kindnesses beyond all expectations. I am so grateful.

In 2016 a dear friend, colleague, and mentor, Ann Johnson, passed away from a rare type of cancer. In 2017 her family, Jim and Elaine Johnson and Katie Lewandowski, endowed the Ann Johnson Institute for Science, Technology & Society (AJI) at the University of South Carolina and put Allison Marsh and me at the helm. Allison and I wanted to create an institute that reflected Ann's values, an institute oriented toward people, before excellence or impact. We believed, with Ann, that excellence and impact are more likely when individuals enjoy what they are doing and feel supported doing it. Our first step in this endeavor was to surround ourselves with Ann's "people" through our initial external advisory board: Suman Seth, Heidi Voshkul, David Brock, Joe Pitt, Katie Lewandowski, and Karen Rader (thank you all). Our second step was to create programs and initiatives that reflected AJI's people-focused orientation. The result has been a growing family across the science and technology studies (STS) disciplines. Most recently this family was extended by the participants in the 2023 inaugural AJI writing retreat, where I not only met a group of kind, supportive, and just brilliant STS scholars, but also finished the final writing of this book. *None* of this—not the writing or the institute or my sanity—would have been possible without my partner in crime and public historian extraordinaire, Allison Marsh, who is far less a colleague than a dear friend. You are *wonderful*.

My family and I live between two continents—my son once said we live in the middle of the ocean. We (all of us) live in Ireland part of the year and then decamp to the United States for another part of it. This is a chosen life, one that we live to support my career in the United States and my husband's career in Ireland. This life, and thus my career and this book, would not be possible without my husband, John Browne. Thank you for supporting this life, for allowing me the freedom to pursue the work I love where and when I want without ever making me feel like my family might be the cost. I think this freedom is rare and precious, and I do not take it for granted. Thank you also to my children, Lucas, Jonah, and Lillian, who cheerfully and willingly live this life with us and trust me not to screw it up. I couldn't keep doing this if you didn't choose to see our life as a privilege instead of a hardship. You are my favorite people *in the world* and I'm so lucky to have you.

The Puzzle

Contemporary medicine is Janus-faced. Evidence-based medicine is one face of it, emphasizing evidence, statistics, and method. Patient-centered care is the other, prioritizing patient experiences, judgment, and values. Government agencies, policymakers, major insurers, and clinicians have sought ways to bring these faces together. This book is about one such approach, what I call patient-centered measurement. Patient-centered measures can go by other names: the somewhat cumbersome "patient-reported outcome measures" (PROMs) or the slightly whimsical "quality of life measures." Although I will sometimes use these names when referring to historical moments or well-established measures, in this book I will typically call these instruments "patient-centered measures." This moniker aptly reminds us of the tension that exists in the roles these measures are meant to fulfill, but also, I think, better describes the hope they are meant to convey.

Patient-centered measurement is the idea that patient perspectives on, for instance, physical functioning or quality of life should play an evidentiary role in determining how effective a drug is taken to be, the degree to which a hospital provides good-quality care, or whether a particular intervention should be funded by an insurer. This idea may sound prosaic, but in fact it's nothing short of revolutionary. Patient-centered measurement treats patient perspectives *on par* with more traditional metrics such as mortality, morbidity, and safety. It says that patient views matter—not as an afterthought, and not only at the bedside, but in the nuts and bolts of creating our evidence base, and thus in macro- and meso-level healthcare decision-making.[1]

What's more, these measures are very popular. They are part of the Food and Drug Administration's (FDA) initiatives (FDA 2009, 2023), the United Kingdom's development of the National Health Service (2023), and Denmark's policy to improve patient care (Egholm et al. 2023). In 2017 the Organization for Economic Co-operation and Development published a ministerial statement, *The Next Generation of Health Reforms*, urging member countries to develop statistical approaches that would allow the assessment and comparability of patient-reported outcomes. It argues that use

Patient-Centered Measurement. Leah M. McClimans, Oxford University Press. © Oxford University Press 2024.
DOI: 10.1093/oso/9780197572078.003.0001

of these outcomes will better equip countries with data on what matters to patients and how well their care is coordinated. Yet despite these policies, initiatives, and recommendations, patient-centered measures present a puzzle. And this puzzle has its source in the Janus-faced nature of medicine. How can measurement, which relies on standardization, represent patients' perspectives, which, if not idiosyncratic are at least various and changeable?

The stakes for this puzzle are high. If we err on the side of standardization and fail to represent adequately an array of patient perspectives, we risk undermining the ethical values of respect, trust, and autonomy that embody patient-centered care. We also risk epistemic values that speak to our knowledge and understanding of patients' perspectives on, for instance, their functioning or quality of life. If we err on the side of idiosyncratic patient perspectives, we risk the practical, social, and institutional values associated with measuring them, and thus incorporating these perspectives into our evidence base. This book aims to solve this puzzle.

I.1. Patient-Centered Measures

Before I say more about how I plan to solve this puzzle, it might be helpful for some if I say a bit about patient-centered measures, that is, what they look like, how they're used, and what varieties they appear in. Patient-centered measures are presented to people with disabilities, patients, and other ill persons as questionnaires. Some patient-centered measures are "generic," meaning their questions apply to a wide range of illnesses, diseases, and disabilities. For instance, the SF-36 (Ware and Sherbourne 1992) is a well-known, generic, patient-centered measure that asks people questions like these:

Compared to one year ago, how would you rate your health in general now?

- Much better now than one year ago
- Somewhat better now than one year ago
- About the same
- Somewhat worse now than one year ago
- Much worse than one year ago

Other patient-centered measures are condition or disease specific, meaning their questions are restricted to people with a particular illness, disease, or disability. For instance, the Incontinence Impact Questionnaire, Short Form (IIQ-7) (Uebersax et al. 1995), asks women questions like these:

Has urine leakage (incontinence) affected your:

	Not at all	Slightly	Moderately	Greatly
Ability to do household chores (cooking, house-cleaning, laundry)?	0	1	2	3
Physical recreation such as walking, swimming, or other exercise?	0	1	2	3

Patient-centered measures are largely designed to measure a construct or latent trait. Although much could be said to problematize the definition, constructs or latent traits are used in this literature to refer to abstract and (currently) unobservable variables such as intelligence, anxiety, subjective physical functioning, or quality of life. Jum Nunnery and Ira Bernstein (1994) have written that constructs reflect a hypothesis that a set of behaviors, say completing household chores independently and taking part in physical recreation, will correlate with one another or respond similarly to manipulation or intervention. But as I'll discuss in Chapter 1, at least in the context of patient-centered measurement, explicit hypotheses are rare.

Constructs can be multidimensional or unidimensional. Multidimensional constructs have several distinct dimensions related to one another under a single conceptual umbrella. For instance, we might think about anxiety as having cognitive and somatic dimensions. When we think of constructs in relation to measurement, multidimensional constructs are typically measured with multiple scales. Take, for example, the SF-36 (above). The SF-36 measures health status (the construct) on eight different dimensions or scales: physical functioning, role physical, bodily pain, general health, vitality, social functioning, role emotional, and mental health. Unidimensional constructs, on the other hand, have a single underlying dimension; for instance, pain is a construct usually taken to be unidimensional. The IIQ-7 (above) is also unidimensional and thus measured on a single scale (Monticone et al. 2020).

When respondents fill out patient-centered measures, they are confronted with a series of questions. In this literature, these questions are often referred to as "items." Although I will usually refer to questions as questions, sometimes it will make sense to call them items. And just as questions are sometimes called items, measures are sometimes called "tests" (even when they aren't what we naturally would think of as a test). I will usually refer to measures as measures, but occasionally it will make more sense to call them tests.

When respondents answer these questions or "items," their answers are scored to provide measurement or "test" scores. Some measurement models, for instance, Rasch and item-response theory, allow for the use of individual scores and population-level scores. Other measurement models like classical test theory only allow the use of population-level scores. When a patient-centered measure is multidimensional, each scale provides a separate score. Sometimes—depending on a variety of considerations—those scale scores are presented separately and sometimes they are aggregated and presented as a single score. The patient-centered literature sometimes refers to outcomes instead of scores. The term "outcome" can mean different things within the (vast) measurement literature. Eran Tal (2016), for instance, argues that an outcome is different from the answers or raw scores on a questionnaire. Respondent answers and raw scores, on his account, are measurement indications. An outcome is inferred from measurement indications in light of statistical and theoretical assumptions; it is an outcome that refers to a value of the construct, not an indication. But "outcome" also refers to a type of measure used to assess the quality of medical care. In this context an outcome refers to the endpoint of some process or the effect of some cause. In this context outcome measures are contrasted with process or structural measures (not indications) (Donabedian 2005). Because patient-centered measures are often used as evidence of the quality of medical care, and because in any case they are developed in this milieu, the use of "outcome" often refers to their status as endpoints or effects (for a criticism of this use see McClimans and Browne 2012).

When I first encountered patient-centered measures, they were paper-based questionnaires that had to be mailed to potential respondents and then returned by post. My job was to digitalize these measures by scanning them into a computer. It was a time-consuming and labor-intensive process. Now, in many countries, patient-centered measures are completed online. You might find them in your online healthcare portal as a part of measuring your baseline quality of life and, over time, the impact of an intervention.

Or they might be on a device that a researcher gives you to fill out at various time-points during a clinical trial. Patient-centered measures are used in a wide variety of contexts from research to regulation to clinical care. But no matter the context of use they share a common purpose: to represent patient perspectives, to give voice to patients' points of view. But patient points of view are various and changeable, and measurement, at least in this context, tends to expect standardization and invariance. Can patient-centered measures fulfill their purpose? The critical social science literature has long worried about the standardization of patient perspectives and experience (Pols 2006; Mol 2008; Luton 2014). Can these measures overcome those worries? Can this book? I hope so. In the next section, I lay out my plan.

I.2. Book Outline

Patient-Centered Measurement is the result of over a decade of collaboration with psychometricians, clinicians, epidemiologists, and health services researchers. It's unique, in part, because my experience with these collaborators has provided me with a philosophical analysis of these measuring instruments from the inside out. The puzzle at the heart of it—how to represent adequately patient perspectives in measurement—regularly lurks in the space that surrounds many everyday measurement problems. Health researchers are aware that a tension exists, but they rarely address it head-on. Instead, they tend to focus on piecemeal methodological approaches to it, some of which I will discuss in the chapters that follow. As I argue, the result of that approach is that patient-centered measures risk forsaking the ethical and epistemic values that make them revolutionary.

Forsaking these values is a genuine problem. It is a problem for patients whose perspectives are potentially co-opted, for the psychometricians, clinicians, epidemiologists, and health services researchers, many of whom get into this research because they believe in the revolutionary nature of these instruments, and for philosophers who have generally ignored or misunderstood the nature of these instruments. What is the solution? *Patient-Centered Measurement* responds with what philosopher's call an "epistemic" theory drawn from what we label the hermeneutic tradition, to show how these instruments can be representative and inclusive of patient perspectives. This solution offers an evaluative practice to hone (not a methodology to follow), and a process through which we can improve the epistemic and moral quality of these measures. Words like "epistemic" and "hermeneutic" have precise meanings in philosophy, but I can explain them simply here. Epistemic simply means related to knowledge, and in this book, it is most usefully contrasted with method. Sometimes methods can give us knowledge, but epistemic investigations, especially in this book, probe the limitations of methods. The hermeneutic tradition—the word derives from the Greek meaning to "interpret"—refers to a discipline and a historical movement that treats the interpretation of texts, human action, experience, measurement as a distinct topic of study (George 2021).

In the first two chapters of this book, I discuss how the health science and philosophical literature have failed to address sufficiently the epistemic and ethical values of these instruments. I begin in Chapter 1 with the health science literature. This literature is fascinating because on one level researchers are aware of the ethical and epistemic dimensions of their instruments, and, what's more, it concerns them. For example, researchers and policymakers extol the ethical virtues of patient-centered measures. Their main ethical virtue? To place patients at the center of questions of evaluation, or, as researchers often say, to "represent patients' perspectives." But they worry about whether their instruments are epistemically up to this task (Browne et al. 2017; Fairclough 2017; McKenna 2011) For instance, in a 2001 article from the *British Medical Journal* titled "Are Quality of Life Measures Patient-Centred?" (Carr and Higginson 2001) the authors wonder whether standardized metrics can genuinely represent patient perspectives. According to Google Scholar this article has been cited over 700 times. In another article, from the *Journal of the American Medical Association*, titled "The Problem with Quality of Life in Medicine" (Leplège and Hunt 1997), the authors argue that these measures cannot represent patient perspectives if patients aren't involved in developing the constructs, for instance, physical functioning or quality of life, used by the instruments. This article has been cited over 800 times.

These concerns, which I label above as "epistemic," are developed in the health science literature as concerns over a lack of theory (Hunt 1997; Hobart et al. 2007). Researchers worry that their constructs are theoretically underdeveloped. Moreover, they worry that this lack of theory development jeopardizes the relationship between the measuring instrument and the construct it aims to measure—the relationship that philosophers refer to as coordination, and psychometricians call construct validity. While I agree that patient-centered measurement faces problems with coordination (or validity), I disagree with this diagnosis. Measurement does not require the-oretically robust constructs to get started. Rather, measuring a construct helps to develop a more theoretically robust construct. For instance, before we had a theory of temperature, early metrologists began measuring temper-ature by bodily sensations of hot and cold. They noticed that fluids expand their volume when heated, which led to theorizing about why; investigation into heat expansion led to the development of new instruments to measure "temperature," which eventually led to the development of fixed points, a numerical scale, and quantification. Each innovation increased the scope of metrologists' theorizing of temperature. This example of temperature not-withstanding, as health researchers attempt to solve what they understand as a problem of theory, they tend to reach for off-the-shelf methods and models as the solution. But, as I argue in this chapter, this solution simultaneously complicates and avoids resolving questions of coordination and validity.

How can we improve the epistemic quality of these instruments and help them live up to their ethical promise? We need to adopt a lesson learned from studying the history of measurement in the physical sciences, namely that coordination in measurement has the structure of a hermeneutic circle (van Fraassen 2008). The upshot of this lesson is we must accept that we do not have access to value-free, assumption-free, in short, infallible evidence of the construct we are interested in measuring or their relationship to our meas-uring instruments. Learning this lesson means embracing a certain amount of uncertainty when we measure and accepting that our methods cannot save us from this fate.

In Chapter 2 I turn from the health science literature to the philosoph-ical literature on well-being. The philosophical literature is almost a mirror image of the health sciences literature—while the health science literature misunderstands the epistemic significance of theory development, the phi-losophy of well-being literature misunderstands the ethical significance of these measures. Philosophers interested in measurement in the social sci-ences tend to assume that the ethical virtue of these instruments is benevo-lence. That is, they tend to assume that the point of measuring, say, physical functioning or quality of life, is primarily to promote policies that will im-prove the well-being of populations. Philosophical theories of patient-centered measures are often taken from the well-being literature and are oriented toward this ethical value.

It may be that benevolence is the main ethical virtue in some areas of meas-urement in the social sciences, for instance, development and economics, but it is not the main ethical virtue in patient-centered measurement. Patient-centered instruments seek to capture patient perspectives and represent patient voices; they are defined by their revolutionary promise to put these perspectives at the center of medical assessment and evaluation. In Chapter 2 I argue that autonomy, not benevolence, best epitomizes the moral impulse of patient-centered measures. Moreover, I argue specifically that patient-centered measures are *patient-centered* to the degree they

1. Prioritize patient involvement
2. Be inclusive of patient perspectives

In Chapters 3 and 4, I explore these criteria and develop over the course of these chapters an epistemic theory of patient-centered measurement. This theory offers a procedural account of patient-centered measurement; a procedural account for how to prioritize patient involvement and ensure inclusivity. This account revolves around two processes:

1. Epistemic dialogue
2. Ongoing coordination

In Chapter 3 I develop my account of epistemic dialogue. Epistemic dialogue spells out what it means for patient involvement to be prioritized. People with disabilities, patients, and other ill persons should be our primary partners in coming to understand patient-centered constructs and developing their conceptual frameworks. Their testimony provides us with invaluable expertise. It does not mean, however, that health researchers should always simply acquiesce to these understandings. On the contrary, health researchers have a responsibility to understand and operationalize patient-centered constructs, and this responsibility requires asking questions and maybe even disagreeing. The testimony of people with disabilities, patients, and other ill persons is invaluable but not infallible.

Here is a preview of my argument. Traditionally, patient-centered measures have been developed by clinicians and health researchers and then applied to populations of patients. This meant—and sometimes still means—that non-patients develop the questions in a measure that they believe are most important to patients with a particular condition, such as epilepsy. Patients then answer these questions, thus providing the information that will form the basis of a claim about the construct. This process of measure development has some fairly obvious problems. It tends, for example, to reinforce identity stereotypes. Here is how it happens. When clinicians and health researchers develop patient-centered measures for people with, for instance, epilepsy, they tend to focus on the frequency and strength of seizures because this is what they think is most important to patients' physical functioning or quality of life. People with epilepsy then answer questions about the frequency and strength of their seizures. This information both (1) forms the basis of a claim about their physical functioning or quality of life and (2) reinforces the claim that frequency and strength of seizures is important to the physical functioning or quality of life of people with epilepsy.

Yet qualitative research involving people with epilepsy suggests that while seizures do affect physical functioning and quality of life, the social stigma of seizures is equally, if not more, important. Moreover, social support seems to mitigate the anxiety of seizures. The questions clinicians and health researchers ask don't reveal the whole picture of physical functioning or quality of life with epilepsy. Moreover, the part of the picture it does reveal helps to reinforce the stigma that seizures are a barrier to a good life. Relying on clinicians and health researchers to develop a measure's questions in the absence of patients is both epistemically and morally problematic. Epistemically, it limits what we can come to know about, for instance, physical functioning or quality of life in a patient population. Ethically, it is grievously unjust to claim that patients' responses to questions are representative of their perspectives when the questions they are answering may reinforce damaging stereotypes, for instance, that people with epilepsy are incapable of employment or have violent tendencies.

The argument I have outlined so far is broadly similar to themes in the health science literature over the previous decade. Across that period, there was an increasing recognition that representing patient perspectives requires patient representation in measure development, that is, findings from qualitative studies from patients should be used to develop a measure's conceptual model, and the questions used in a measure. Thus, patient-centered instruments should prioritize patient involvement. This requirement has been widely embraced, by the FDA, the International Society for Pharmacoeconomics and Outcomes Research (ISOPOR), and assorted textbooks (FDA 2009; Rothman et al. 2009; de Vet et al. 2011). Yet this point is still important to make because while the health science literature recognizes the importance of involving people with disabilities, patients, and other ill persons in measure development, the philosophical literature, as I will discuss in Chapter 3, has lagged.

In addition to this point about the philosophical literature, it's important to discuss epistemic dialogue in patient-centered measures because epistemic dialogue goes beyond the idea about taking the testimony of people with disabilities, patients, and other ill persons seriously. Epistemic dialogue is not simply a glorified version of qualitative research. Rather epistemic dialogue goes beyond qualitative research and the recommendations from the FDA and ISOPOR. It says that just as we must take seriously first-person illness experiences, we must also take seriously the secondhand points of view from health researchers, clinicians, and others who have a stake in these instruments. They too have expertise relevant to the development of patient-centered measures. To be sure, their expertise isn't expertise of what it is like to have a particular disability, condition, or illness, but it is still important. Measure development should develop practices and norms that allow health researchers, clinicians, people with disabilities, patients, and other ill persons to engage with one another. If this sounds like pie-in-the-sky philosophy, it isn't. But you'll have to wait for Chapters 3 and 4 to be convinced.

In the development of epistemic dialogue, I conceive of people with disabilities, patients, and other ill persons as partners with health researchers and clinicians in developing patient-centered measures. That is, I conceive of them as having a development role vis-à-vis patient-centered measures. In Chapter 4, I consider people with disabilities, patients, and other ill persons in their role as respondents, as people who answer the questions posed in these measures. In doing so, I address the second criterion for patient-centeredness: inclusion. Let me set the stage by sketching out the problem. Even when people with disabilities, patients, and other ill persons contribute to measure development through epistemic dialogue, it is still the case that the meanings they give questions and answers will change over time (longitudinally) and at a single point in time across individuals (cross-sectionally). In other words, even when we do our very best to create measures with questions that are sensitive to the experience of respondents, these questions won't resonate (or won't resonate in the same way) with all respondents for all time. In a nutshell: patient-centered constructs, and the questions that address them, are context sensitive. If we want our measures to be fit for purpose—valid and fair—then we must respond to at least some of these changes in meaning. In other words, we need to ensure our measures are more inclusive of diverse patient experiences. Yet the questions in these measures are designed to be standardized, not only in their wording but also in their meaning.

So how do we create more inclusive measures? Ultimately, my answer is that patient-centered measures must have ongoing coordination. But to motivate this answer it's useful to begin with some of the literature on what has been termed "responses shift," or changes in the meaning of a patient's evaluation of the target construct (Sprangers and Schwartz 1999). In the late 1990s some of the health measurement literature started to recognize that constructs such as quality of life, physical functioning, and mobility can have different meanings for different people. The idea that patient-centered measurement has a responsibility to reflect these different meanings is expressed through the literature on individualized quality of life measures (Joyce et al. 1999). These measures forgo attempts to standardize a construct across a population and instead tailor each measure's questions to a particular respondent. The spirit of this concern is advanced through contemporary work on response shift. Unlike individualized quality of life, response shift is often explored in the context of standardized measures. Response shifts are often most visible when a patient responds to the same questionnaire at two or more points in time. Consider, for instance, a person who reports extensive limitations in pursuing leisure activities after one round of chemotherapy, but three months later, after five rounds of chemotherapy and with worsened health, reports only mild limitations. These answers suggest that quality of life for this person has improved while health has worsened. Examples such as this one have perplexed health researchers. Are response shifts a form of measurement error? Or do they represent important information about respondents' quality of life?

Response shifts are similar in some ways to what philosophers refer to as adaptive preferences. Arguments that explain away changes in preference as merely adaptive tend to assume that the cause of the adaptation, for instance changes in health state due to cancer or disability, is bad (Barnes 2016). But why should we accept this assumption when patients tell a different story— they report that quality of life can improve or remain the same even when health or ability changes. Moreover, if response shifts are the result of changes that radically affect respondents in epistemic and personal ways, experiences that L. A. Paul (2014) has called transformative, then it's difficult to know how those of us without the relevant experience can judge the authenticity of patient responses. In fact, I argue we should not try. We should instead have an inclusive approach, taking patient responses seriously even if (especially if) respondent answers surprise us. This means accepting, in principle, the legitimacy of response shifts and applying their insights to our measurement models.

In Chapter 4 I examine two interpretations of what response shift is and how to model it. I examine the "appraisal account" (Schwartz and Rapkin 2004; Rapkin and Schwartz 2004) and the principle of conditional independence (PCI) account (Vanier et al. 2021). I argue that, of the two, the appraisal account is better at distinguishing response shift from measurement error. The PCI account says that violations of PCI indicate response shift when observed scores on repeated administrations of a test are not independent of the time of the test (or individual characteristics that change with time) (Oort et al. 2009). What does this mean? It's helpful to start with PCI. In the context of patient-centered measurement, PCI is fulfilled if given knowledge of, say, physical health, the scores on a test for subjective physical functioning are invariant for, say, gender. Intuitively, considering the physical health of our sample population, this means that knowing their scores on the test tells us nothing about their gender, and knowing their gender tells us nothing about their scores. Violations of PCI that indicate response shift occur when test scores are not invariant with respect to change over time; that is, something about the time between test administrations affects the measurement results.

The appraisal account says that whenever we answer questions, we use a set of cognitive processes to determine the meaning of a question. These cognitive processes are things like establishing a frame of reference (Were you limited in pursuing your leisure activities *with respect to gardening*?) and standards of comparison (Were you *now as opposed to five years ago* limited in pursing your leisure activities?). Appraisal metrics (Rapkin et al. 2017, 2018) help to measure differences in how respondents understand questions on a patient-centered measure. They provide the *backstory*, if you will, about what is going on when respondents answer questions. Appraisal metrics thus help to interpret respondents' measurement scores and make them more clinically meaningful.

To be sure, not all instances of appraisal are also instances of response shift. Response shifts are essentially unexpected changes in appraisal. But being able to identify response shifts via appraisal is useful because it aids in *coordination*. Coordination refers to the process by which we link measuring processes with constructs. It's through coordination that we can have confidence in a measurement value's being a value of a specific construct (instead of something else entirely). Appraisal gives us insight into how respondents understand questions and answers and thus whether their scores meaning-fully refer to the construct as it was conceived. Because response shifts will occur, we must anticipate that our measures will lose coordination over time or among different populations. Consequently, measurement coordination is not one and done; it is ongoing. Information from appraisal can feed into coordination in at least two ways. We might use appraisal information to ad-just our interpretation of measurement outcomes for some subpopulation. Alternatively, we might alter patient-centered measures themselves to better reflect respondent understandings (or avoid them), or we might re-define the construct of interest—perhaps splitting it into two constructs or reconceptualizing it altogether.

Moving on from Chapters 3 and 4, where I lay out my theory for patient-centered measures, in Chapters 5 and 6 I discuss possible challenges to it. In Chapter 5 I take up the question of measurability of patient-centered constructs, and in Chapter 6 I discuss the pharmaceutical industry's poten-tial to exploit the patient-centered focus I give these instruments.

Are constructs such as physical functioning and quality of life measurable? If this question is posed to psychometricians or philosophers of science, the answers, whether yes or no, will most likely involve a discussion of measure-ment scales and whether interval-level representation is justified. Since I dis-cuss some of these concerns in Chapter 1, in Chapter 5 I set them aside and focus instead on the implications of this question when posed to philosophers of well-being. In the well-being literature, philosophers tend to think of measurability in terms of *heterogeneity* (Hausman 2015; Alexandrova 2017). Heterogeneity is the idea that the goods required to make one individual's life go well are sufficiently different from those required to make others' lives go well. If the goods required for a good life are different for individuals, then measuring a good life is difficult. When you combine heterogeneity with a desire to create measures that are sensitive to individual perspectives, some philosophers of well-being conclude that these constructs aren't measurable, or if they are measurable, it's only in a limited way.

In this chapter I compare three different accounts of heterogeneity: Dan Hausman's (2015) account in *Valuing Health: Well-Being, Freedom, and Suffering*, Anna Alexandrova's (2017) account in *A Philosophy for the Science of Well-Being*, and Bruce Rapkin, Caroline Schwartz, and colleagues' account across a number of papers. I argue that all three of these accounts concep-tualize heterogeneity as a barrier to measurement; that is, if we are able to measure well-being or quality of life, it's despite heterogeneity. For instance,

Hausman and Alexandrova agree that constructs like well-being and quality of life are heterogeneous. For the purposes of using these measures to direct policy, Hausman thinks they are too heterogeneous: Alexandrova disagrees. She argues that if we focus on disease and condition-specific measures, which she calls contextual well-being, then we can eliminate much of the heterogeneity that makes them problematic. Schwartz et al. (2020a), on the other hand, locate heterogeneity not in patient-centered constructs, but in the perspectives of respondents. If this distinction makes sense (and I argue that it doesn't), it has the benefit of keeping patient-centered constructs homogenous.

Contrary to these approaches, I argue if we can measure patient-centered constructs at all it's because of heterogeneity, not despite it. In making this argument I help myself to some lessons from the philosopher Hans-Georg Gadamer's writings on hermeneutics. The upshot of these lessons is that while it's possible to talk abstractly about "constructs" and "subjective perspectives," it's only through the application of perspective to constructs that we have something we can meaningfully study, investigate, probe, or *measure*. In other words, it is only when respondents answer questions about patient-centered constructs that we have empirical content at all. The price of having patient-centered content that we can investigate and measure is that it comes to us as heterogeneous material because respondents will often answer questions differently from one another and differently over time. But of course, I don't think this is much of a price because (1) patient-centered measures are an important force for good and (2) we can manage heterogeneity with creative applications of appraisal metrics and ongoing coordination.

In Chapter 6 I turn to a problem with patient-centered approaches and pharmaceutical industries. Recently philosophers have discussed how these commercial concerns can co-opt and exploit approaches to incorporate patient perspectives into drug development (e.g., Holman and Geisler 2018; Bueter and Saana 2020). For instance, pharmaceutical companies have sponsored patients to attend FDA patient-focused drug development meetings. The concern is that industry is using the FDA's interest in patient perspectives to capture the discussion at these meetings and further its own economic interests rather than the interests of patients. Do patient-centered measures play into the hands of industry? Here is the issue. My account of patient-centered measures emphasizes the importance of taking the testimony and responses of people with disabilities, patients, and other ill persons seriously regardless of "race, religion or creed." Might this approach to equality open these measures up to exploitation? Moreover, my counterweight to some of these concerns is epistemic dialogue, a form of critical dialogue oriented toward achieving a better—more coherent—understanding through the give-and-take of questions and answers. But might this approach also be open to capture?

One alternative to taking all patients equally seriously and relying on epistemic dialogue is to discount the testimony of some patients based on, for instance, their funding or other concerns regarding how they might distort expressions of needs and values or misdirect goals (Warnke 2014). This alternative is what Georgia Warnke (2014) calls "pulling rank." We might pull rank on some patients because we distrust their testimony for one reason or another. I argue against this alternative for patient-centered measurement, and I argue for further dialogue instead. This isn't to say that patient-centered measures aren't open to capture or something similar. In this chapter I offer two examples of how these measures are vulnerable to industry's economic interests. Yet I also argue that in these cases industry's ability to manipulate patient centered measures is largely due to its success in obscuring questions of values (harms and benefits) and economics (profits and losses) while highlighting a narrow version of scientific rigor. This interest in a particular representation of scientific rigor benefits pharmaceutical industries.

Instead of pulling rank, I argue, we ought to change the conversation to include questions of values and economics rather than limit it. In the end, both pulling rank and promoting further dialogue have their risks. But epistemic dialogue avoids the risk of silencing and ignoring patients who should be heard—and who's to say whose testimony is worthwhile and whose isn't? History is littered with examples of getting this wrong. Pulling rank, moreover, risks exacerbating power plays and turning attention away from the things that matter, things like improving healthcare decision-making and making it more responsive to human needs. Although I recognize the desire to pull rank, it is not the appropriate response to patient-centered measures: we double down on dialogue.

I.3. Guide for the Reader

This book tells a story about patient-centered measures, with each successive chapter building on the next. At the same time, the chapters have been developed in pairs with each twinset encompassing a theme. Chapters 1 and 2 discuss misconceptions of patient-centered measures, first from the context of the health sciences and then from the philosophy of well-being. Chapters 4 and 5 lay out my theory of patient-centered measures, explaining how epistemic dialogue prioritizes patients and ongoing coordination achieves inclusion. In Chapters 5 and 6, I examine challenges to my theory: measurability and industry exploitation. Readers particularly interested in one or more of these themes can pick up these chapters out of order. A final note: about half way through writing this book I bought a horse and then . . . a pony. Examples and stories of my adventures pepper these chapters beginning with Chapter 4, so if you love horses you may want to start here.

PART I
MOVING AWAY
FROM STANDARD ASSUMPTIONS
Health Science and Philosophy

1

Coordination, Validation, and the Hermeneutic Circle

What is quality of life with urinary incontinence? Or subjective functioning after a spinal cord injury? Or more generally, what is quality of life in the context of health-related conditions? Neither philosophers nor health researchers have settled answers to these questions. Yet it is common in the context of healthcare, evidence-based medicine, and evidence-based policy to make claims about a population's health-related quality of life using what I refer to in this book as patient-centered measures. But if we don't know what we're measuring, how can we make epistemically grounded claims about it? For over two decades this problem has worried an increasing number of health researchers and philosophers. In this chapter I argue we don't need settled answers to these questions to make justified claims (which is good because we don't have them and maybe never will). But we do need to recognize the assumptions and implicit values we bring to these questions, and we need to be open to the ways our assumptions and values may be wrong. Put otherwise, we don't need theories of quality of life; instead, we need a hermeneutic approach to the practice of measurement.

In everyday life and in science we are often in the position of acting under conditions of uncertainty. Most of us are aware of the ethical difference between those who acknowledge uncertainty and proceed with humility, and those who ignore uncertainty and proceed with confidence. Under conditions of uncertainty mistakes are always possible. You might mistakenly identify one thing as another. You might give people bad advice on which they act, thus causing harm to themselves or others. Under conditions of uncertainty, what goes wrong in these cases isn't merely epistemic. When there is a limit to what we can know for sure, justification must turn to ethics. Was proper attention given to what was unknown? Were the risks of being wrong (to oneself and others) properly considered (Biddle and Kukla 2017)? Were the merits of alternative points of view and courses of action contemplated?

Patient-Centered Measurement. Leah M. McClimans, Oxford University Press. © Oxford University Press 2024.
DOI: 10.1093/oso/9780197572078.003.0002

There is a word for people who make claims beyond their sphere of knowledge: ultracrepidarian. The problem with ultracrepidarians is not that they make epistemic mistakes, but rather they make mistakes due to puffed up overconfidence. I think the worry that undergirds the concern that we don't know what quality of life *is* (Hunt 1977; Leplège and Hunt 1977; Carr and Higginson 2001; Hobart et al. 2007), is, perhaps, that claims made by patient-centered measures about physical functioning or quality of life are ultracrepidarian. Perhaps patient-centered measures make claims that go beyond what can be justified. And maybe when they do, it indicates hubris on the part of those making the claims. Much of this book can be understood as a story about avoiding this kind of hubris in the context of patient-centered measurement. In this chapter, I discuss how we might justify measurement claims about quality of life and other patient-centered constructs even when we are uncertain about all these constructs entail. To do this I look at examples from the history of science and hermeneutics. I argue that justifying our measurement claims requires facing up to what we don't know about the constructs we wish to measure. Facing up to what we don't know, I further argue, means grappling with what is called the hermeneutic circle (I'll explain that term in a minute) that characterizes measurement. In the second half of this chapter, I examine contemporary attempts within patient-centered measurement to justify claims about their constructs, and find these attempts lacking. Rather than grappling with the hermeneutic circle, these attempts too often sever it.

1.1. Validity

The way we talk about validity, what we think validity *is*, has changed over time (Edwards et al. 2018).[1] In the mid-20th century validity tended to be understood as a property of an instrument; for instance, a measure was considered valid or not. But in the last 30 years or so validity has come to be understood as the property of an argument about the evidence supporting the use of measurement outcomes or test scores. In the patient-centered measurement literature both usages continue to prevail. Health researchers use validity to mean different things and communicate with this term in what Peter Galison (1999) calls trading zones.[2] These are highly localized spaces that allow scientific subcultures within the larger culture to communicate and share knowledge despite disagreeing on definitions or classification schemes. I will generally consider validity to be the property of an argument about the use of outcomes, but when referring to the use of validity in specific studies, documents, or subcultures I will follow their usage, which in some instances refers to validity as the property of a measure.

If we lack evidence for the validity of patient-centered outcomes for a particular use, then the numerical values derived from the measure may not adequately represent the construct in that context. Invalid arguments for the use of outcomes can have serious consequences. Consider: patient-centered measures are usually classified as "outcome measures" (for a criticism of this classification see McClimans and Browne 2012). That is, they are designed to reflect the impact of a service or intervention on a patient-relevant construct such as physical functioning or quality of life. As such, patient-centered outcomes are sometimes used as evidence for resource allocation decisions, drug approvals, and claims of clinical effectiveness; for instance, we might use patient-centered measures as evidence of the clinical effectiveness of conservative surgery versus mastectomy following early detection of breast cancer. If we lack validity evidence, a measure's claims can undermine the fair allocation of resources, honest drug labeling claims, and decisions about what is the right treatment to recommend. These claims can materially impact marginalized populations via clinical recommendations, insurance funding, and pharmaceutical marketing. Consider an example. Patient-centered measures are sometimes applied to populations and individuals to describe their disease burden or monitor individual progress. In this capacity, patient-centered outcomes are used to judge how populations or individuals are doing with a particular disease, disability, or illness. Judge wrongly and this can have far-reaching social, emotional, and economic consequences.

Researchers sometimes worry that because we don't have settled answers to questions about what quality of life or physical functioning *is*; we lack sufficient validity evidence and contribute to the harms discussed above. This worry gets expressed in two related ways:

1. Constructs such as physical functioning and quality of life are not well understood
2. Measurement results are not well understood

Health researchers tend to be particularly concerned with the first problem. They tend to explain why constructs are poorly understood in terms of a "lack of gold standard." For those who use this explanation, it serves to explain why they believe theory is important to these measures. "Lack of a gold standard" means patient-centered measures lack external criteria against which measurement results can be compared and interpreted. Think of the answer key to a math exam. This is a gold standard. It can be used to judge student answers as correct or incorrect, rank student exam results, and provide them with meaning. It also defines the construct under measurement, for example, mathematical aptitude. Patient-centered measures don't have an answer key. When asked about my general health compared to a year ago, I might say, "About the same." Who's to say I'm wrong? To be sure, sometimes there are incorrect answers; for instance, if I am perfectly able to get myself in and out of the bath but when asked whether I can do it, I answer no. But, regardless of this example, after administering a questionnaire, third parties often won't know if an answer is correct or not. This uncertainty is part of what leads researchers to conclude: we don't know what quality of life is.

In a 1997 editorial, "The Problem with Quality of Life Research," Sonja Hunt (1997, 206) diagnosed the lack of a gold standard as the primary problem with quality of life measurement; she referred to it as the "crux" of the matter. This absence is used by Hunt and others to explain certain features of patient-centered measures. For instance, David Streiner and Geoffrey Norman (2003, 178) in their book *Health Measurement Scales* link the need to validate the degree to which patient-centered instruments represent the constructs they aim to measure with their lack of observable content. Jeremy Hobart and colleagues (2007, 1095) allude to the lack of a gold standard to explain why patient-centered constructs must be measured indirectly via questions instead of directly, like the way we measure height. For her part Hunt (1997, 206) connects this absence to (1) the dubious validity of patient-centered measures, and (2) problems interpreting their outcomes, that is, determining their clinical significance.

For these researchers the lack of a gold standard leads to complications for validity. Their reasoning, which Hunt (1997) helps render explicit, is that criteria external to a measure would help form a consensus regarding the meaning of constructs such as quality of life. According to Streiner and Norman (2003, 178), observational criteria are available when we measure height and weight, but not when we measure psychological constructs. In their view, theory is important in lieu of a gold standard because if we can't see the constructs, then theory is needed to direct us to the manifestations of them. They write:

Attributes such as height or weight are readily observable, or can be "operationally defined"; that is, defined by the way they are measured. . . . Once
we move away from the realm of physical attributes into more "psychological" ones like anxiety . . . we begin dealing with more abstract variables,
ones that cannot be directly observed. We cannot "see" anxiety; all we can
observe are behaviours which, according to our theory of anxiety, are the
results of it. (2003, 178)

Regarding the second problem above, that is, the difficulty understanding
measurement results, Denny Borsboom (2005, 71) writes, "For most test
scores we still have no idea whether they really measure something, or are no
more than relatively arbitrary summations of item responses." This second
problem is a reflection of the first: if the construct is not well understood,
we won't have good predictions about how a measure should function. If
we don't know what to expect from the measure, then we don't know if the
scores represent the construct or not. They could just be, as Borsboom writes,
"arbitrary summations." The problem of understanding a measure's results
is sometimes cashed out in the health measurement literature as "interpretability." Interpretability refers to the clinical as opposed to statistical meaningfulness of the scores produced by the instrument. For instance, if cancer
patients tend to improve by about 10 points on the Treatment of Cancer
Quality of Life Questionnaire (EORTC QLQ C-30) over the course of three
months while receiving a new form of treatment, we would like to know what
this improvement means. Are they able to enjoy more hobbies? Socialize
more regularly? (McClimans 2011). But if we don't know enough about the
construct and how it is represented on the scale, then these inferences are difficult to make. Indeed, interpreting the scores of patient-centered measures
has proven difficult, and this in turn has limited their usefulness, particularly
their clinical usefulness.[3]

As we saw above, health researchers who worry about validity tend to think
the solution to this problem is *theory*. For over two decades health researchers
have lamented the lack of theory in patient-centered measurement, as Hunt
did in her 1997 editorial. In 2009, the late Professor Donna Lamping's pres-
idential address to the International Society for Quality of Life Research
(ISOQoL) enumerated the need for a theoretical framework as one of three
challenges facing the field. In 2019 the leadership of ISOQoL sought ways to
emphasize theory in the discipline.[4] Philosophers and psychometricians also
agree: these measures need theory (Alexandrova 2017; Hobart et al. 2007;

Borsboom 2006). Although there are differences among proponents about what sort of theories are required, there is a general, if abstract, consensus that theory improves validity by improving knowledge of the construct and generating predictions about instrument behavior.

For readers familiar with the philosophy of measurement, the juxtaposition of the two problems above may be familiar. Philosophers of measurement, like health researchers, worry about the connection between unobservable entities they wish to measure and the measuring instruments that aim to measure them. This worry continues in the natural sciences despite well-developed physical theories in which these entities figure. In the philosophy of measurement literature this worry about the connection between entities and instruments is referred to as the coordination problem. In Bas van Fraassen's discussion of the problem, he frames it as a question of imbuing physical theories with empirical significance, or, as he writes, "understanding how scientific theory is more than its mathematical guise" (2008, 115). For van Fraassen, it's usually through measurement that theories acquire empirical support, so coordination becomes a question of how measurement can establish the value of what is measured. As we've seen, health researchers, who have typically lacked robust theories of their constructs, tend to focus on imbuing measurement scores with theoretical substance. But it is telling in this initial comparison with the natural sciences that the worry about coordination, or validity, persists in the natural sciences even in light of well-developed theories. If these questions persist, then perhaps theory isn't what we need to secure coordination. In the next section I discuss the coordination problem in more detail, taking up a case study from the history of science. I argue that in fact we don't need well-developed theories to measure temperature, physical functioning, or quality of life; rather we need to grapple with the hermeneutic circle in which measurement resides. We will move away from the concrete questions of health measures for a brief period in order to understand the broader philosophical issues involved. Don't worry: it will soon be clear why working through the history of philosophy is a necessary digression toward a solution of our problem.[5]

1.2. Measurement and the Hermeneutic Circle

The coordination problem presents a puzzle. Imagine I'm studying the quality of life of people with irritable bowel syndrome (IBS). To further my research,

I decide to use a quality of life measure in my study—this measure will help me to understand better what quality of life with IBS means within a certain population. I apply this measure to a sample of people who have IBS. I get the results back. I now find myself asking, "Is this a good measure of quality of life for people with IBS? Does it accurately reflect their quality of life?" It might be a good measure, but I'm not sure because I don't know enough about quality of life with IBS to anticipate how the construct should behave when measured. But now we are back to where I started before I applied the measure: "What does quality of life with IBS look like?" Establishing validity for patient-centered measures confronts a circle. This is the connection between the problems I discussed above, that is, understanding constructs and understanding the scores on a patient-centered measure.

In his discussion of the coordination problem, van Fraassen (2008, 116) argues that coordination has the structure of a circle—a hermeneutic circle. In considering coordination from the point of view of physics, he argues that answers to the questions, "What counts as a measurement of X?" and "What is X?" presuppose one another. In other words, theorizing about duration, temperature, or quality of life isn't done in isolation, but rather involves measurement. Similarly, measurement doesn't occur in isolation, but anticipates theory. For instance, if I am theorizing about quality of life with IBS, part of doing this is developing a hypothesis and testing it. Measures are an integral part of testing predictions. On the other hand, the process of creating a test and choosing a measure to investigate my prediction is a process that must be tailored to my understanding of quality of life with IBS. Yet, if van Fraassen is correct about the hermeneutic structure of coordination, how does measure development or theory development get off the ground? Moreover, how can we tell if our measures and theories are justified instead of mutually reinforcing prejudice and bias? To answer these questions, it's helpful to get a grip on the hermeneutic structure that van Fraassen (2008) argues characterizes coordination.

The basic idea of the hermeneutic circle is there is no understanding—no knowledge—without presuppositions (Grondin 1997). All knowledge rests on assumptions. The hermeneutic circle is traditionally conceptualized in terms of a relationship of parts to a whole. The canonical example of this relationship is a text, but hermeneutics has also been applied to a host of other topics, including human action, jurisprudence, social science, medicine, and, by means of van Fraassen, measurement. But let's take up the example of a text. Reading a text faces the same conundrum as coordination in measurement. We come to have knowledge of a text as a whole only in virtue of already understanding something of its parts. But we understand parts of a text only in light of a general understanding of a text as a whole. How do we ever get started? For me, nothing illustrates the hermeneutic circle better than my first encounter with European philosophy, which happened to be the German philosopher Martin Heidegger's *Sein und Zeit* (hereafter *Being and Time*). I couldn't get beyond the first page (it had one paragraph). I had no idea what to make of the sentences. It was an English translation. I could read them aloud. Yet I had no idea what they might mean. But how could I? I had no previous experience with this kind of philosophy, no general understanding of what the text could possibly be about. In sum, I had no "whole" from which to make sense of the parts. I spent a long time in the dark, but as Professor Dwight Furrow began to explain bits and pieces to me, and I continued to muddle through that first page, I finally got a better sense of what the first few paragraphs *might* be about. This understanding of one part of this complex text allowed me to project a more general understanding of the whole, which in turn helped me to understand further sections of it. Applied to measurement, we might say we understand a particular construct when we know how to anticipate its behavior through measurement. Yet we understand how to anticipate a construct's behavior only when we understand the construct.

If you hold the view that scientific knowledge should be objective in virtue of being assumption or value free, then van Fraassen's (2008) claim that co-ordination in measurement is circular will seem problematic. Hermeneutics, as I describe above, only gets started once we can muster some coherent assumptions. Indeed, as Jean Grondin (1997) writes, classic hermeneuticists strove to avoid the hermeneutic circle and the presuppositions that, in their view, tainted objective knowledge. Nonetheless, 20th-century hermeneuticists such as Heidegger, Ricœur, and Gadamer have viewed the circle as productive of knowledge, and in any case inescapable. Contemporary philosophers of measurement seem to concur. In addition to van Fraassen (2008), Hasok Chang (2004) also discusses the circularity involved in justifying measurement in *Inventing Temperature: Measurement and Scientific Progress*. Over the course of four case studies, Chang (2004) argues, in a fashion surprisingly similar to Gadamer's work in *Wahrheit und Methode* (1960/2004) (hereafter *Truth and Method*), that empirical science cannot escape circularity. Chang's (2004) solution to the coordination problem is what he refers to as coherentism. I discuss the similarity of Chang's and Gadamer's work in what follows.

1.2.1. Coherentism and Philosophical Hermeneutics

The likeness between Chang (2004) and Gadamer (2004) is perhaps partly explained by the parallels found in their philosophical antagonists. In *Truth and Method*, Gadamer (2004) is reacting to an account of hermeneutics that relativizes the meaning of a text to the historical or biological conditions under which the text is written. The idea here is that we often misunderstand texts, as well as one another, because we interpret them from a particular vantage point, one that is historically conditioned by presuppositions and values. Behind this idea is a worry. If we can only understand a text or one another through historical presuppositions and values, then how do we prevent the hermeneutic circle from simply repeating the mistakes of the past? For example, how do we forestall sexist or ableist interpretations from reinforcing sexist and ableist presuppositions and values? Put otherwise, how can we use our understanding of empirical studies or human action to change or enrich our presuppositions and values? How, in other words, does our understanding progress?

One answer to this question is to sanitize understanding and interpretation from presuppositions and values. To this end, classical hermeneuticists argued for a rigorous methodology focused on the motivations under which texts and actions originate. The aim of this approach is to secure our hermeneutic foundations against what Gadamer (2004) calls "effective history." If we can have done with historically conditioned presuppositions and values, then understanding no longer progresses in a circle, and the threat of it turning vicious is neutralized.

In *Inventing Temperature*, Chang (2004, 221) reacts to an account of justification in the natural sciences that seeks a self-justifying foundation as the evidence base for the empirical sciences. The primary benefit of such an evidence base is that it appears to safeguard scientific knowledge from presuppositions and values. He refers to this position as empiricist foundationalism. Like methodological hermeneutics, which I discuss above, empiricist foundationalism seeks to secure scientific knowledge from presuppositions and values. The worry behind this solution is also similar. If scientific knowledge claims are not insulated from presuppositions and values, then how do we know if our knowledge claims are founded or unfounded? Put otherwise, how can we justify our belief in certain claims when we know that the presuppositions and values affecting them are fallible? Moreover, what stops pseudoscientific claims from reinforcing a pseudoscientific worldview? How do we know if scientific knowledge is progressing or digressing? As with methodological hermeneutics, empiricist foundationalism's answer is to purify scientific knowledge from presuppositions and values, thus denying the relevance of these questions.

We can all agree that knowledge and understanding are threatened by a vicious circle of part and whole, measurement no less than anything else. The solution put forward by classical hermeneutists and empiricist foundationalists, however, is not realistic. We cannot anesthetize assumptions and values. They are as much responsible for knowledge and understanding as they are a cause of concern (Gadamer 2004). Consider again the examples I gave of reading *Being and Time* and interpreting the measurement results of quality of life with IBS. There is no meaningful way forward with this text or measure unless we have some idea of what they might be about—epistemically, normatively, aesthetically. Without these kinds of assumptions and values the opening paragraphs of *Being and Time* and the results from patient-centered measures are simply words and numbers on a page ("arbitrary summations"). They have no meaning. Meaningfulness requires that we fit these words and numbers into a larger whole in which we already know our place. Yet the necessity of assumptions and values for understanding doesn't mean we can we simply ignore the demands of justification (see Chang 2004, 222–23). If we cannot escape the hermeneutic circle, then we should turn our energies to ensuring the circle is productive or, as we might say, "virtuous." Chang (2004) shares this ambition with Gadamer (2004).

In contrast to empiricist foundationalism, Chang (2004) argues that his case studies in the development of thermometry offer historical evidence for a coherentist approach to the justification and progress of scientific knowledge. Rather than a self-justifying evidence base, early temperature metrologists made do with the, admittedly, fallible knowledge they had at the time, in order to ask questions and develop strategies to drive thermometry forward. But how did they do it? How does Chang's coherentist approach avoid vicious circularity?

Two features characterize Chang's coherentist framework. It is conservative and it is pluralistic. These characteristics are not unique to accounts aiming to work within the hermeneutic circle. Gadamer's (2004) hermeneutics shares Chang's (2004) conservativism, and Gadamer's most careful interpreter, Georgia Warnke (1999), extends his work to embody a similar pluralism. The plural aspect of these accounts stems from the recognition that with different theoretical and practical commitments, as well as different historical and cultural standpoints, we can learn different, yet equally legitimate, lessons from the same topic. The conservative aspect of these accounts is the consequence of rejecting attempts to sanitize knowledge. If we cannot break free from the part-whole relationship through self-justifying beliefs or rule-bound methodologies, then we have no choice but to recognize our historically conditioned position within the hermeneutic circle: a position that is rife with assumptions that are the result of historically effected interpretations. This recognition means acknowledging that our epistemic position is full of imperfections handed down to us through history. Chang (2004) refers to this acknowledgment as the principle of respect.

Chang is not particularly clear in explaining why respect is the attitude we should cultivate. Given what we know about the history of science, and the sexist, racist, ableist and other values that have enabled at least some of it, one might wonder if skepticism might be a better attitude. Gadamer (2004), in his discussion of the rehabilitation of authority and tradition, however, provides an explanation for Chang's choice. In this section of *Truth and Method* Gadamer reacts to the Enlightenment's antithesis of reason versus authority and tradition. He argues that this is a false dichotomy. Tradition does not proceed without reason, nor is reason free of tradition. To be sure, we are born into a historical tradition, and this tradition exerts an authority over us insofar as it orients us into the world. We are, as Heidegger (1927/1996) puts it, "thrown beings." But, as Gadamer (2004) and Heidegger contend, our "thrownness" does not mean we cannot use reason, albeit historically situated reason, to question our tradition and change its course. Nor does tradition "persist because of the inertia of what once existed" (Gadamer 2004, 281). Rather, traditions need to be "affirmed, embraced, cultivated" through reasoning with others about them (Gadamer 2004, 281).

Chang's use of respect in relation to the affirmation of a knowledge system, seems to refer to the space wherein we reason about a tradition and find it useful. Respect, then, denotes the proper attitude toward an existing knowledge system that one deems imperfect, but still beneficial. Indeed Chang (2004, 231) emphasizes that scientists can choose the knowledge system they affirm, and chafes against Thomas Kuhn's (1977) suggestion that such systems are inherited within particular scientific disciplines. I want to leave to one side the question of how many degrees of freedom scientists have in making such choices, and instead assume minimally that Gadamer and Chang agree at least this much: given the right conditions, we can create space between the tradition we are born or educated into and our ability to critically reflect on it.

Although coherentism begins with respect, the "driving force" of its progress, as Chang (2004, 44) refers to it, is epistemic iteration. Put otherwise, epistemic iteration is Chang's rebuttal to those who worry about vicious circular reasoning. Chang (2004, 226) defines epistemic iteration as "a process in which successive stages of knowledge, each building on the preceding one, are created in order to enhance the achievement of certain epistemic goals. In each step, the later stage is based on the earlier stage, but cannot be deduced from it in any straightforward sense." One example Chang uses to illustrate this process is the development of temperature standards. Early metrologists working within the principle of respect affirmed bodily sensations of hot and cold as a necessary starting point for standardizing temperature. But their understanding of temperature did not remain limited to what the body can detect. Their understanding was not viciously circular. Instead, using bodily sensations as a reference point, they noticed that fluids change their volume when heated and cooled. Investigation into these volume changes led to the development of thermoscopes, a tube through which one can view the rise and fall of a liquid with changes in temperature.

Thermoscopes afforded metrologists a standard more accurate than bodily sensation by which to observe temperature changes, and with them they were able to observe a larger range of phenomena. By refining thermoscopes and their use of them, metrologists were eventually able to judge which fluids were sufficiently constant when heated and cooled to function as fixed points. Once metrologists were able to fix two points, it became possible to develop a numerical scale, which made way for the next evolution: the quantification of temperature. Quantification allowed for mathematical calculations about temperature, which, Chang (2004, 48) explains, paved the way for theorizing about thermometric observations. When it became clear that the fixed points first employed were not as fixed as metrologists had believed, they advanced their understanding of temperature through strategies to fix existing points and through the use of new fixed points.

This very brief discussion is meant to illustrate the progressive advances of successive iterations of temperature standards. The lesson Chang (2004) intends to convey is that beginning with imperfect assumptions does not doom us to repeat them. Yet we are left with questions. Even if the circle is not vicious, how do we know it is progressive? How do we know our knowledge about a topic is better, more illuminating, or less reliant on invalid assumptions? How, in other words, can we be sure that we haven't simply discarded one set of invalid assumptions and replaced them with another invalid set? Chang's (2004) response is twofold. First, knowledge claims are valid, or we might say justified, when they belong to a system of mutually supportive beliefs—when they are coherent with other beliefs. Second, our progress should be measured in terms of whether a system of knowledge has furthered any of its epistemic virtues. Philosophers have long noted multiple epistemic virtues such as simplicity, fertility, and testability.

For Chang, knowledge is justified and progressive when it is coherent with other beliefs and furthers epistemic virtues. This means that scientific progress embodies a certain amount of pluralism. As he (2004, 232–33) puts it: "The methodology of epistemic iteration allows the flourishing of competing traditions, each of which can progress on its own basis without always needing to be judged in relation to others." Epistemic iteration is different from relativism because the coherentism Chang advocates is evaluated in terms of progress toward epistemic virtues. Our scientific beliefs must be coherent with respect to our other beliefs, but they are also tested in terms of their simplicity, fertility, testability and so on.

As I discussed earlier, Chang's (2004) arguments on scientific justification and progress in the natural sciences echo Gadamer's (2004) discussion of interpretation and understanding in the social sciences. But Gadamer and his contemporary interpreters (for instance, Grondin 1997, 2003 and Warnke 1999, 2011) seem to take more seriously the question of misunderstanding. At any rate they give a more thorough account of it. Above I asked how we know that the epistemic iterations are progressive. How do we know that our knowledge in a successive iteration is better and less reliant on invalid assumptions? Chang's response is that iterations must be coherent and enhance a range of epistemic values. Gadamer, on the other hand, focuses on one particular epistemic virtue that Chang eschews: "possible truth." Using the idea of possible truth, Gadamer argues that we should assume in advance that a text or its analogue is valid or, put differently, that it has something to teach us. To put a contemporary spin on this point: we must practice epistemic humility (Ho 2011).

We might read Gadamer as saying that one of the conditions of understanding requires reasoning about the historical tradition handed down to us. But the space for this reasoning only opens when we are pulled up short by a text, when our assumptions and values snag in their ability to make sense of a text. Being pulled up short by a text creates a space where we can recognize our assumptions and values *as* assumptions and values, as part of a historical tradition that could be wrong. We prepare to be pulled up short—to reason about our assumptions and values—by adopting a humble attitude, by assuming a text has something to teach us. For Gadamer, we have much to learn from texts and from others, and part of this recognition is accepting the possibility that we can be wrong. Possible truth requires us to take a text and others seriously. For Gadamer possible truth is an important counterweight to the historically conditioned assumptions and values we bring to any text.

Gadamerian hermeneutics is a back-and-forth between the assumptions and values we bring to understanding—our tradition—and the possible truth that an encounter with a text or its analogue may bring to our understanding. We might think of this back-and-forth as hermeneutic reasoning between the past (our tradition) and the future (new ways of understanding). For Gadamer it is because we assume a text or its analogue has something to teach us that we can gain access to assumptions and values we did not know we had. For instance, in quality of life research one surprising finding that I will discuss in later chapters is that physical health can get worse while quality of life self-reports improve. This phenomena is sometimes referred to as "response shift". If I treat the improvement in quality of life as possibly true, then a space opens for me to reflect on how this result might be true and why I find it surprising. This helps me to detect and crucially evaluate an assumption that I may not have known I held: namely, quality of life is indexed to physical health. Once this assumption is laid bare, I can ask whether it is reasonable given results from other quality of life studies, but also other things I know about the world. One thing I know about the world is that humans are marvelously adaptable. This adaptation, however, may give me pause in detaching quality of life from physical health. There are some situations to which humans should not have to adapt; where adaptation suggests false consciousness. At the same time there are contexts in which claims to false consciousness are thinly veiled paternalisms. This back-and-forth of hermeneutic reasoning allows me to test and revise my assumptions—to earn respect for the tradition—while also investigating new understandings and their place in the whole.

In Chapter 3 I will have more to say about Gadamer's proposal that we take a text to be possibly true. For my current purposes, it is enough to illustrate that the hermeneutic circle need not be vicious. Chang and Gadamer, philosophers from two very different philosophical traditions, nonetheless come to similar conclusions. The hermeneutic circle can be productive, and what's more, it cannot be avoided if we wish to justify knowledge claims and validate our measuring instruments. Measures and texts, it turns out, are more similar than we may have thought. In both cases we must reconcile parts and whole. As I discuss above with the example of quality of life and response shift, projected understandings of a construct help us to understand measurement results, and in turn measurement results help to refine our understanding of a construct. Just as projected understandings of what *Being and Time* might be about help to make sense of the opening paragraphs, readers who continue to muddle through these paragraphs will use this understanding to clarify the text as a whole. Moreover, both texts and measures are open to multiple interpretations. In fact, in Chapter 4 I'll discuss, in an extended example, two different interpretations of response shift results and their different impacts on our understanding of patient-centered constructs.

In the next section I return to patient-centered measures to investigate what happens when, similar to methodological hermeneutics and empiricist foundationalism, measurement theories strive to neutralize the effect of untested assumptions and values about the construct of interest. I'll argue that neutralizing assumptions and values stymies the growth and potential of patient-centered measures. Specifically, it inhibits validity and coordination.

1.3. Measurement Theory

As I discussed earlier, health researchers and others have sometimes suggested that lack of theory is responsible for questions about the validity of patient-centered measures. Yet concerns about coordination persist in the natural sciences despite well-developed theories of the quantities being measured. Moreover, measures of temperature existed before well-developed theories did (Chang 2004). Although theory plays an important role in science for many reasons, coordination does not seem to require it. My discussion in the previous section suggests that while coordination doesn't require a theory, it does require coherent assumptions about a construct (or theoretical entity), and this might also include what we sometimes refer to informally as "theorizing." These assumptions are projections that by their nature go beyond what we *know* about a construct. Thus, for Gadamer, the counterweight to these assumptions is the possible truth that confronts us in the form of, for instance, measurement results or testimony from people with disabilities. Treating measurement results and testimony as true doesn't just serve as a *check* on our assumptions, it also helps to *illuminate* assumptions. This last point is important because we can't reason about assumptions that we don't know we have.

If van Fraassen (2007) is correct that the questions "What is X?" and "What counts as a measure of X?" presuppose one another, then the existence of patient-centered measures suggests some notion of what they measure. To be sure, we may not, on reflection, agree with the assumptions implied by a particular measure, but this disagreement is the point of the exercise. It indicates a moment when we can reason about a measure as well as other beliefs we may have about a measure's construct. This reasoning process is in fact the story of epistemic iteration. Thus in lieu of readily available construct theories or perhaps readily accessible assumptions about patient-centered constructs, measures might, in principle, be a good place to begin when developing validity arguments. Nonetheless, I'll argue that instead of using measures as a way of *generating* assumptions to begin epistemic iterations, measurement theories such as classical test theory and Rasch measurement theory serve to repress them.

1.3.1. Classical Test Theory

How do researchers justify the inference from the answers respondents provide on patient-centered measures—what Tal (2016) calls measurement indications—to outcomes that express a knowledge claim about a construct of interest, for instance, quality of life or physical functioning? Health researchers attempt to justify the inference using measurement theories such as classical test theory and Rasch measurement theory (Wilson 2013). In this section I discuss CTT and in the next I discuss Rasch.

Although CTT has roots in the 19th century through the development of laws of error and true scores, it embodies three main ideas that have a foothold in the 20th century: first, the recognition of error in measurement, second, the idea that error can be conceptualized as a random variable, and third, the notion of correlation and how to index it. The development of CTT begins in 1904 with Charles Spearman's demonstration of how to correct a correlation coefficient due to measurement error, and reaches maturity with Melvin Novick's discussion in 1968 (Traub 1997). CTT turns on a simple model where the expected value of observed scores (O), that is, the empirical data acquired after someone fills out a questionnaire, is equal to a person's true score (T) plus uncertainty, commonly termed random error E, thus O = T + E.

When using CTT the value of the true score is taken to be a theoretically unknown value, which is assumed to be constant, and the expected observed score is assumed to be a random variable that produces a bell-shaped curve around the true score. The error score is taken to have an expectation value of zero. The idea here is that as the number of observations increases, that is, administrations of the questionnaire increase, the random errors will tend to cancel one another out; thus the mean of the observations is taken as an estimate of the true score. To acquire an empirical value for T in the context of patient-centered measurement, a person must be measured repeatedly on a scale (fill out a questionnaire), and each observation (individual questions or repeated administration of the same questionnaire) must be independent of the others (Hobart and Cano 2009).

In some contexts, using CTT makes sense. Borsboom (2005, 14–15), following Adolphe Quetelet's work (see Porter 1985), provides an example from astronomy. Imagine that we want to locate the position of a planet that is far enough away that its position can be considered constant. We take multiple careful measurements, but they do not yield identical results. We can interpret the deviations in measurements as random error, for instance, the result of weather, shaky hands, etc. Moreover, in this context such measurements usually produce a bell-shaped curve around the true score. But in the context of the behavioral sciences, CTT makes less sense.

First, unlike the position of a distant planet, repeated administrations of a questionnaire are not independent of one another. Respondents remember the questions from previous administrations and re-evaluate their answers in light of them. Second, patient-centered measures do not function as a "series of repeated measurements" (Borsboom 2005, 15); rather, they function as "measurements on a single occasion" (Borsboom 2005, 15). In a series of repeated measurements, the true score should remain the same from one administration of the questionnaire to another. But patient-centered measures do not function in this way. Apart from the fact that respondents will remember their answers from previous questionnaires, it is also the case that patients' health can change over the course of administrations of the questionnaire. Indeed patient-centered measures are often employed precisely to measure change over time. Third, the interpretation of the observed score as an estimate of the true score significantly depends on the assumption of a continuous variable, for example, distance, with a normal probability distribution. But many of the variables in the context of patient-centered measures are categorical rather than continuous, as the responses elicited from respondents to individual questions can take only a limited number of values, for instance, strongly agree, agree, disagree, strongly disagree.

These difficulties, as well as others, are well known (Borsboom 2006; Cano and Hobart 2011). Typically, the first two are managed through a thought experiment: imagine the person filling out the questionnaire is brainwashed between a series of administrations (Lord and Novick 2008). This thought experiment renders administrations of a questionnaire independent of one another and enables us to interpret the administrations as a series of measurements. The third difficulty is often dealt with by simply ignoring the categorical nature of the data elicited from individual questions and assuming that the variable approximates continuity given a large-enough number of possible values that can be derived from combinations of responses to different questions.

When CTT is put into practice, the model reduces to O = T. CTT is, thus, what I call a "permissive" measurement theory. If the point of a measurement theory is to justify the inference from measurement indications to outcomes, then CTT appears to justify every inference with equal credibility—any instrument with an observed score also has a true score, that is, has a measurable construct. Regardless of where you come down on the value of CTT to patient-centered measurement, it lacks an important epistemic virtue: testability.[6]

We can trace the problem with CTT to the theory of errors in which it is situated. Within this theory, the idea that random errors will cancel one another out in the long run, that is, the error score will have an expectation value of zero, is an empirical assumption (Borsboom 2005). The hypothesis that an observed score estimates the true score is contingent on this empirical assumption. But, in the context of patient-centered measurement, there are no empirical grounds for making this assumption since (1) patient-centered measures are not correctly understood as a repeated series of measurements; and (2) they are not independent of one another.

1.3.1.1. CTT and Validation

At the beginning of Section 1.3 I said that measurement theories such as CTT and Rasch serve as different justifications for inferring from a measure's indications to an outcome of interest. Colloquially, these theories should justify why we should believe that respondent answers shed light on quality of life as opposed to something else. Yet CTT does not provide insight into the specific construct an instrument measure. At most, CTT tells us that our indications refer to *something* we can measure. Another way to put this point is that CTT does not model the relationship between an observed score and the construct of interest (Borsboom 2005; Hobart et al. 2007; McClimans 2011). Here is the first place where CTT serves to sever the hermeneutic circle.

We might ask, why is the true score not an estimate of the construct of interest? In the context of CTT, true scores are relative to a particular measuring instrument: every instrument with a mean observed score has a true score. Yet, in practice, quality of life researchers don't take this proliferation of true scores to imply that every measuring instrument targets a different construct. They are not operationalists in this sense. Even after researchers use CTT, they still ask if, or to what degree, the instrument measures the construct it is meant to measure. Researchers rely on validity tests, not true scores, to determine if an instrument measures the intended construct (Streiner and Norman 2008, 247–76).

So what is construct validity? The literature on this topic is complicated. In fact, Borsboom (2006) refers to construct validity as a "black hole from which nothing can escape." The problem is not that the methodology of construct validity is complex, but rather the sheer diversity of questions that construct validity is meant to answer, and the varieties of tests used to determine it make it complicated to untangle. Indeed, as I discussed toward the beginning of this chapter, what we take to be validity has changed over time (Edwards et al. 2018). Discussions that parse out construct validity from other forms predate current trends that treat validity wholistically. Nonetheless, these validity distinctions persist in the patient-centered literature and are part of my discussion in this section.

To simplify this exploration of construct validity in CTT, I refer to Lee Cronbach and Paul Meehl's classic 1955 article on the subject. They argue that construct validation is used when what is meant to be measured is not "operationally defined" (Cronbach and Meehl 1955, 282); that is, construct validity is needed when we lack a criterion or consensus on the content of what is to be measured. The question that construct validity poses refer us back to the coordination problem: what counts as a measure of x when we are unsure of what x is. In the context of CTT, the question about construct validity is usually answered with tests of convergent and discriminant validity because they are typically taken to provide the most robust evidence.[7] Broadly speaking, convergent validity testing is used when researchers believe a dimension or scale from one instrument should correlate with a dimension or scale from a comparator instrument. Discriminant validity testing is used when researchers think a dimension or scale from one instrument is relatively unrelated to a dimension or scale from another instrument.

To apply convergent and discriminant validity tests, specific hypotheses are supposed to be formulated regarding the kind of similarities or differences anticipated between the validating and comparator instrument. This emphasis on hypothesis formation makes sense given the stress on theory development discussed earlier. Nonetheless, these hypotheses are rarely created (Abma et al. 2016). I'll discuss this dearth of hypothesis development and its effect on validity later. For now, it's enough to note the process through which construct validity is, at least in principle, established. For both convergent and discriminant validity, comparator instrument(s) are chosen, and this instrument along with the instrument being validated are applied to a sample of respondents. The true scores from these instruments are then correlated. If the hypotheses are correct given these correlations, then these correlations contribute to the evidence that the instrument being validated measures a similar or dissimilar construct from the one to which it is being compared. This is intended to be an iterative process: the more hypotheses tested, the stronger the evidence of validity (Abma et al. 2016). In Cronbach and Meehl's (1955, 290) language, convergent and discriminant validity testing helps to elaborate the nomological network of the construct(s) of interest. A nomological network is a theory that comprises a set of laws that link theoretical representations of the construct(s) being measured along with their observable manifestations.

Classic and contemporary descriptions of construct validity in patient-centered measurement almost always begin with the need for a theory or hypothetical model of the construct of interest (e.g., Cronbach and Meehl 1955; Streiner and Norman 2003; Fayer and Machin 2007). It's from this theory or model that hypotheses are meant to be developed when testing for convergent or discriminant validity. Perhaps this prevalence is not surprising given, as I discussed above, the penchant to think theory will solve questions about validity. Nonetheless, the very same articles and textbooks that emphasize the need for theory are evasive about the content of these theories or where such theories can be found. Indeed, the nomological nets envisioned by Cronbach and Meehl did not come to fruition (Schimmack 2021). But without theories or hypotheses, how are patient-centered measures construct validated in practice?

In practice, correlations between the instrument being validated and the comparator instrument are correlated without the use of hypotheses. But this answer raises another question: Without hypotheses, what are the grounds for accepting a particular correlation as evidence of construct validity? This question is not widely discussed in the literature. Nonetheless, the lack of hypothesis generation in validity testing did rise to the level of awareness in the development of the Consensus-Based Standards for the Selection of Health Measurement (COSMIN) (Mokkink et al. 2010). COSMIN is an initiative to help health researchers, policymakers, and clinicians select the correct patient-centered measure for research and clinical practice. COSMIN relies on convergent and discriminant validity evidence to help make measurement selections, but without hypotheses to ground these tests the evidence they provide is questionable. COSMIN thus developed generic hypotheses that could be applied to convergent and discriminant validity tests. These generic hypotheses provide standard criteria that COSMIN reviewers can use to evaluate the methodological adequacy of construct validation studies when the authors of these studies don't generate their own hypotheses (Mokkink et al. 2010, 41). Here are the generic hypotheses used by COSMIN:

1. Correlations with (changes in) instruments measuring similar constructs should be ≥.50.
2. Correlations with (changes in) instruments measuring related, but dissimilar, constructs should be lower, that is, .30–.50.
3. Correlations with (changes in) instruments measuring unrelated constructs should be <.30.

Recall that methodological hermeneutics and empirical foundationalism sought to safeguard knowledge by anesthetizing assumptions and values through self-justifying beliefs and rule-bound methodologies (see McClimans and Browne 2011). Similarly the standardized hypotheses developed by COSMIN also have the appearance of safeguarding knowledge by anesthetizing assumptions and values. A measure can be construct validated without hardly mentioning the construct in question. Yet to apply the standardized hypotheses, health researchers, policymakers, and clinicians must determine the appropriate level of correlation hypothesis. This determination requires a judgment regarding how similar or different an instrument is from the comparator instrument, and this in turn requires some assumptions about what it is that both instruments measure, and why they should be similar or different. Yet, because these assumptions are un-articulated, they go unrecognized, unchallenged, and untested. Indeed, part of Gadamer's (2004, 270) criticism of methodological hermeneutics is that those who do not acknowledge the assumptions and values at work in their own understanding are still dominated by them. To be sure, some construct validation studies don't use COSMIN's hypotheses, but unless the correlations found in construct validation studies are used to illuminate rather than silence the assumptions that brought the validating and compar-ator instruments together, my criticism remains the same.

I am not the first to notice the lengths to which psychometricians and those working on patient-centered measures go to avoid engaging with the constructs they aim to measure (Alexandrova and Haybron 2016; Alexandrova 2017). I suggest that this avoidance is similar to methodolog-ical hermeneuticist's and empirical foundationalist's efforts to secure knowl-edge from presuppositions and values. Yet, as I will discuss at more length in Chapter 3, Gadamer is correct that ignoring our assumptions and values does not secure us from their influence. When non-patients, non-disabled, and non-ill people design the questions that populate patient-centered measures, their assumptions about illness and health can prejudice the instruments.

I have argued in this chapter that theories are not prerequisites for devel-oping patient-centered measures. Rather developing a measure is like writing a book, and books do not need well-developed theories before an author puts pen to paper. But authors do need to know something about the topic they wish to develop in a book. Authors do research in their topic. They have ex-plicit and implicit assumptions about it. If writing is always historically con-ditioned, writers can prepare themselves to be pulled up short, sometimes by their own writing, sometimes by unexpected insights into their topic. As authors work to create parts that will turn into a coherent whole, they must keep asking questions about their topic. They must engage with the topic even though what it *is* is a moving target, even though their engagement is imperfect. The same kind of questioning, of engagement, is necessary for measure development, including validation. Just as it's important for authors to grapple with their topic of interest, so too should measure developers ac-knowledge, articulate, and question the constructs they aim to measure. But it is just this kind of engagement with the construct that is generally missing in construct validation studies. The lack of hypothesis generation that caused

COSMIN to develop generic hypotheses is telling, not because it speaks to the need for theory to replace them, but because it illustrates a lack of engagement with the constructs being measured.

Psychometricians recognize the limitations of CTT (Hobart and Cano 2009; Rusch et al. 2017; Smith et al. 2019; Petrillo et al. 2014). Yet the majority of psychological measuring instruments, including patient-centered measures, are based on it (Borsboom 2006; Hobart et al. 2007; Wilson 2013). The popularity of CTT is not due to a lack of other available measurement theories. Latent trait theories (also known as modern test theories to distinguish them from classical test theory) such as Rasch measurement theory, which I discuss in the next section, and item response theory, offer alternatives. Rather, the popularity of CTT lies, I suspect, partly in its simplicity. What CTT lacks in testability it makes up for in its easy and forgiving nature. In the context of an undertheorized field, CTT offers a lot of leeway. Situated within a theory of errors, CTT doesn't require researchers to theorize itemized sources of error, and situated within a simple model, there are fewer restrictions on the structure the data must exhibit for the construct to be deemed measurable.

1.3.2. Rasch Measurement Theory

In this section, my primary purpose is to evaluate Rasch measurement theory as an alternative answer to the coordination problem. But in the psychometric literature, Rasch is best known for its relation to fundamental measurement. To better evaluate Rasch as an answer to the coordination problem, as well as its limitations, a short introduction to fundamental measurement and Rasch's relation to it is useful.

The Rasch measurement theory was first described by Georg Rasch (1960), a Danish mathematician who argued that the core requirement of measurement in the behavioral sciences should be the same as that in physical sciences. In making this comparison with the physical sciences, Rasch joins Norman Campbell (1920) and others such as David Krantz, Duncan Luce, Patrick Suppes, and Amos Tversky (1971) in focusing on measurability and scale development. For Rasch, measurable attributes must be quantitative variables, and measurement is the identification of values of these variables, that is, the creation of measurement scales. Accordingly, for a variable to be measurable (quantitative) it must be structured such that the values of the variable stand in certain algebraic relations to one another. Specifically, the relations must be ordered, that is, transitive, and additive (conforming to the properties of addition, e.g., commutativity). Depending on the structure of a variable, it may or may not be measurable. For example, whether or not depression is measurable will depend on whether its values stand in the right relation to one another; the answer to this question plays out in the data from questionnaires.

Campbell (1920) argued that measurement procedures are additive and thus fundamental when their values can be derived by concatenation. To take a well-worn example, it is possible to establish an interval measurement scale for length given (1) the qualitative difference in the length of, for example, single rigid rods, and; (2) the concatenation of two or more rods with another set (Krantz et al. 1971). Unfortunately, attributes from the behavioral sciences (and indeed some from the physical sciences) do not permit concatenation operations. In 1964, however, Luce and Tukey argued for a new type of fundamental measurement, which does not require concatenation: additive conjoint measurement. Conjoint measurement is a process that provides evidence (or not) that a psychological construct or latent trait is quantitative. Conjoint additivity thus opens the possibility of fundamental measurement and interval-level scales for the behavioral sciences. Although Rasch models (Rasch 1960) predate Luce and Tukey (1964), some have argued that they are a form of additive conjoint measurement (Keats 1967; Brogden 1977; Perline et al. 1979).[8]

Those who favor Rasch measurement theory for patient-centered measures usually do so because they see it as holding the key to establishing interval-level measurement in this field. How does Rasch work? Rasch models the probability of a right or wrong response to an item (question) as a function of a person's ability and a question's difficulty. Rasch presupposes (1) that a person with greater ability should have a greater probability of answering an item correctly, and (2) that given two items one of which is more difficult than the other, a person has a greater probability of answering the easier question. Given these relationships, Rasch models can establish measurement values for person ability and item (question) difficulty.

Rasch models are based on a logistic function. Scales produced by these models use the logit as a measurement unit, that is, the logarithm of the odds that a respondent makes a correct response. The formula for one variant of the Rasch model for items with dichotomous response options is the following:

$$Pr\left\{x_{ni}|\beta_n,\delta_i\right\}=\frac{e^{x_{ni}(\beta_n-\delta_i)}}{1+e^{(\beta_n-\delta_i)}}$$

where the likelihood of a person n answering an item i correctly is $x_{ni} \in [0,1]$; β_n and δ_i are the measurements of the ability of person n and the difficulty of item i, respectively, upon the same latent trait, and e is the natural logarithm constant (2.718). In applications of Rasch to patient-centered measurement, these models often concern levels of severity or frequency on a rating scale interpreted as indicating more or less health, disease burden, functionality, engagement in decision-making, and so on.

The extent to which patients' responses to questions (the data) "fit" the predictions of those responses from a Rasch model, within acceptable uncertainty, is the extent to which measurement is achieved, that is, the extent to which we can infer interval-level data. Put otherwise, Rasch models help us to pick out those questionnaires that measure a quantitative construct. To be sure, we still don't know anything substantive about the construct it measures or the meaningfulness of the way the items cohere. All we know is the measurement scale we can apply to the construct. For those who believe interval-level scales are necessary to measurement, this is a big step forward.

1.3.2.1. Rasch and Validation

The Rasch model's ability to produce interval-level measurement is usually what is emphasized in the literature. But do Rasch models aid in coordinating constructs with empirical content? Do they provide an answer to the coordination problem? Do Rasch models help us to understand better what, for example, physical functioning is, and whether our instrument measures it?

Rasch is more restrictive than CTT in terms of what questionnaire data it deems measurable. Rasch measurement theory provides a hypothesis about what the empirical data of a construct should look like. Unlike CTT, which outsources hypothesis formation to construct validity, Rasch takes some of this responsibility on for itself. Consequently, Rasch is testable. Measurement indications may or may not be consistent with a Rasch model; that is, the empirical difficulty of the items may or may not be consistent, unidimensional, invariant, and so on, across the persons and items measured. If not, then for those who take the Rasch model to be a standard of measurement, the construct in question is not measurable. On the other hand, if the questionnaire data do fit the model's predictions with acceptable uncertainty, then we've gained information about the difficulty of our items and the ability of our respondents. This informational gain, plus the interval-level scale, improves the interpretability of Rasch instruments compared to CTT ones. Rasch thus allows us to get some grip on the relationship between measurement data and the construct we want to measure. In other words: Rasch does facilitate certain kinds of inferences from measurement indications.

Nonetheless, a Rasch model by itself does not underwrite an inference from measurement indications to the measurement outcome, for instance, physical functioning. To make this inference, we must have a Rasch model in conjunction with a construct theory. In this respect Rasch measurement theory is similar to CTT. When questionnaire data fit a Rasch model's predictions, what we have is a linear scale or "ruler" on which items with increasing difficulty and persons with increasing ability go in one direction, and decreasing difficulty and ability go in the other. But from the point of view of the model, the content of the items that fill out the ruler are a black box; that is, the model doesn't care if the questions refer to getting in and out of the bath independently or walking on an uneven surface. Both CTT and Rasch measurement theory give us information about the measurability of a construct, yet they are typically not used to generate assumptions about the construct itself. And as I will argue, when it comes to the content of the construct, the practical application of Rasch can be as theory avoidant as CTT.

Determining the validity for a Rasch measure is a two-part process. Both parts need to be completed to underwrite an inference from an instrument's indications to the outcome of interest. The first part is a question of fit; that is, do the questionnaire's item-level data fit the predictions of a Rasch model within acceptable certainty to support useful inferences about ability and difficulty? The second part concerns the substance of the construct: Does the empirical item order conform to our understanding of the construct, for example, do the questions at the difficult end of the ruler make sense? (Wilson 2005; Stenner et al. 2013).

It is reasonable to expect that in the second part we would compare the empirical item order in the first part to a set of assumptions about what that order ought to look like, or we might use the item order to raise assumptions and thus questions about that order—as I've been arguing, we need not have a full-blown theory. But the second part of the validation process often collapses into the first. Consider an example. In the ABILHAND questionnaire for upper-limb manual ability in patients with rheumatoid arthritis (RA), extensive research with RA patients and experts in the field developed an item pool of 56 questions. A subsequent Rasch analysis reduced the pool to 27 items ordered from least difficult (picking up a can) to most difficult (opening a jar) (Durez et al. 2007). At this point validity testing requires researchers to ask how the 27-item Rasch ordering compares to the larger set of questions from the qualitative research. Ideally, researchers would use the larger set of items to challenge the smaller set, to raise questions about it and thus ultimately strengthen the justification for the ordering. For instance, in the development of the ABILHAND, items such as "buttoning up a shirt" and "counting banknotes" failed the statistical tests of fit to the Rasch model and were discarded (Durez et al. 2007). But there is no discussion or explanation of the discard apart from their failure to meet the demands of the Rasch model.

In the discussion section of the paper the authors rationalize the item order that emerges from the data. They do this by comparing the results obtained from patients with RA to patients who have suffered a stroke. Here again, this comparison might have been used to generate questions. Instead, the RA ordering is taken for granted:

> When compared with the items retained in chronic stroke patients, it is striking that (1) more unimanual activities have been retained in RA and (2) some activities are perceived with different difficulty in both diseases. For instance, three activities are more difficult for patients with chronic stroke because they involve greater bimanual coordination (wrapping up gifts, filing one's nails and cutting meat) and two are more difficult for patients with RA because they generate higher mechanical constraints in the upper limb joints (taking the cap off a bottle, fastening a snap-fastener). (Durez et al. 2007, 1102–3)

The assumption that guides the justification of included items in the ABILHAND is the general constraint imposed by the Rasch model; that is, ability and difficulty should be mathematically related. The justification for discarding items is misfit with the Rasch model. To be sure, this one example doesn't generalize to all those who use Rasch to develop patient-centered measures. Sometimes the item ordering following the Rasch analysis does lead to questions about why an item received the difficulty it did or why an item didn't fit the Rasch model. When these questions proceed—all the better. Indeed, discarding items simply because of misfit with the Rasch model is a discredited approach (Bohlig et al. 1998; Stenner et al. 2013).[9]

Yet as the ABILHAND studies illustrate, it is far from an extinct approach. Instead, we often wait for construct theories that are slow to materialize and focus attention on the Rasch model.

1.4. Conclusion

The point of measurement theories such as CTT and Rasch is to underwrite inferences from a measure's indications to the construct of interest; to coordinate measuring instruments and what they measure. Both CTT and Rasch, however, often fail to do so because they don't engage with the construct of interest. I started this chapter by arguing that questions of validity and the coordination problem address the same puzzle—and they do, at least in theory. But we've seen that in practice CTT and Rasch cleave questions of validity from the coordination problem. Health measurement textbooks continue to discuss construct validity in terms of providing evidence that an instrument measures what it is meant to measure, that is, evidence of coordination. Yet in the hundreds of validation studies published to provide this evidence, the point is simply to establish correlations with other instruments (CTT) or emphasize the fit of the Rasch model. This is how the two issues are split apart: in practice "validity" merely refers to correlation studies, while at the same time lip service is given to establishing a deeper sense of validity, one that shares the same puzzle as coordination.

To be sure, understanding how one measuring instrument relates to other measuring instruments is necessary information. Moreover, establishing an interval-level scale is an important psychometric and clinical advance. Indeed, knowledge of how instruments relate to one another and to scale development is part of contemporary metrology (Eran 2011; Chang 2004). But none of this is sufficient to *coordinate* patient-centered instruments with the constructs they aim to measure. Without access to the assumptions that ground CTT's correlations, they are empty; without assumptions about the construct a Rasch model measures, claims to validity are unfalsifiable. Although there are hundreds of patient-centered measures that make a claim on validity, most of these claims do not also provide a solution to the coordination problem. In fact, they perpetuate and complicate the problem.

In Section 1.2 I argued that the coordination problem has the structure of a hermeneutic circle; the basic idea here is that there is no knowledge without presuppositions. In discussing Chang's (2004) and Gadamer's

(2004) responses to the hermeneutic circle I emphasized the elements of conservativism and pluralism their accounts share. These elements, I believe, indicate an important, undeniable fact about hermeneutic reasoning. When we enter the hermeneutic circle—and Gadamer would argue that we are always already within it—we find ourselves standing on shifting ground. We must begin from our standpoint or knowledge system knowing that it is imperfect, knowing that some of what we take to be true will be replaced. Moreover, we inevitably face challenges to what we believe in the form of competing accounts, and we must respond to these challenges knowing that our standpoint will inevitably be altered. It is a messy process without any guarantees.

CTT and Rasch seek to avoid this mess through the terra firma of their measurement models. But we saw in Section 1.3 that these models and their respective methods can take us only so far. Eventually they crap out and we are left with quiet, nearly silent assumptions that often make the construct comply with the structure provided by the measurement model. There are two epistemic problems with this approach. First, as I've already indicated, we lose the opportunity to coordinate measurement indications with a construct—we lose the opportunity to learn about what we're measuring. Second, the assumptions made when acquiescing to the measurement model, whether acknowledged or not, affect what is being measured. In fact, when these assumptions are not articulated and evaluated, their effect is more difficult to track. We are more likely to become ultracrepidarian—more inappropriately confident, less appropriately humble—in our inferences about measures.

In the case of Rasch, the effective assumptions go beyond that of an interval-level scale. Rasch models require a standard ordering of items by difficulty across all the persons of interest, within pre-specified statistical boundaries. This requirement ignores that most constructs related to health are a complex interaction of disease processes and the heterogeneity of individual life histories. Without the check of construct engagement, Rasch models erase this complexity.[10] Rasch also moves patient-centered measurement from the realm of patient experience to performance. Rach models conceive of respondents as having more or less of the construct in question, and of the instrument as a test designed to locate respondents' performance. Whether this is the appropriate way to conceptualize patient-centered measurement is an open conceptual question that is made invisible by the acquiescence to the measurement model. Likewise, CTT tends to rely on clinical assumptions to motivate judgments of similarity between a comparator instrument and the instrument awaiting validation. Yet clinical assumptions sometimes assimilate poor health with poor quality of life. As I will discuss in Chapters 3 and 4, these assumptions negatively affect how we interpret measurement indications.

Philosophers and other researchers have long noticed the lack of theoretical engagement in psychological measures. Some have argued (Boyer et al. 2014) that this is due to social scientists' unease with the normativity inherent in the constructs they wish to measure. Others have argued that the problem resides in the relatively separate spheres in which psychologists (who develop theories) and psychometricians (who develop measuring instruments) work (Wilson 2013; Borsboom 2006). Alexandrova (2017, 146) suggests it harkens back to psychologists' operationalist heritage. I think there is something correct in each of these assessments, but in this chapter, I offer a complementary perspective: the problem is not simply a lack of theory, but a refusal to accept the hermeneutic structure within which these instruments must function if they are to mature.

2

Vehicles for Patient-Centered Care

It is not always clear what patient-centered measures assess. As I discussed in the previous chapter health researchers tend to characterize this problem as originating in the lack of a gold standard, and they tend to see a solution in theory development. Yet, despite this characterization, patient-centered constructs continue to lack theory development. Instead, we find what philosophers have referred to as "theory avoidance" (Alexandrova and Haybron 2016). I argued in Chapter 1 that construct theories are not needed to develop patient-centered measures, but I also argued that we cannot avoid engaging with the constructs we hope to measure. While we don't need theories to develop patient-centered measures, we do need to acknowledge the hermeneutic structure in which these measures function. This means explicitly engaging with the constructs we hope to measure; talking about them, questioning them, and revising our instruments and our concepts of them as we learn more. In Chapters 3 and 4 I develop an account of what this engagement of learning and revision might look like. In this chapter I continue to think about the role of theory, but this time from the perspective of the philosophy of well-being.

In the previous chapter I offered CTT and Rasch as examples of measurement models that enable construct avoidance. But if we turn from health measurement to philosophy, we find a much longer tradition of engaging with constructs such as well-being. For those who look to theory to save patient-centered measures, philosophical theories of well-being have often held promise. In this chapter I evaluate two different philosophical approaches sometimes discussed in conjunction with patient-centered measures: subjective well-being and objective list theory. Although these approaches have some obvious merits, I nonetheless argue that they fail to capture what is at stake in patient-centered measurement. And what is at stake? The answer, I suggest, is patient-centeredness itself.[1] To make my concern more explicit, in the first half of this chapter I discuss the historical development of patient-centered measures. Out of this discussion, I posit two requirements for patient-centeredness: (1) prioritize patient involvement and (2) be inclusive

Patient-Centered Measurement. Leah M. McClimans, Oxford University Press. © Oxford University Press 2024.
DOI: 10.1093/oso/9780197572078.003.0003

of patient perspectives. These requirements serve to illustrate what is lacking in subjective well-being and objective list theories and point the way forward toward an account of *patient-centered* measurement.

2.1. Development and Historical Sketch

The developmental history of patient-centered measurement is important if we want to understand these instruments and fruitfully engage with researchers to improve them. In what follows I provide a historical sketch of patient-centered measures to illustrate the central role that patient-centeredness plays in their development.

2.1.1. Emergence of Quality of Life

In his article "Just give me the best quality of life questionnaire: The Karnofsky scale and the history of quality of life measurements in cancer trials," Carsten Timmermann (2013) discusses the first performance scale. Introduced in 1948, the Karnofsky Performance Scale is generally taken to be the first medical instrument to expand assessment beyond physical or clinical dimensions (Fayers and Machin 2000). It was developed to assess how nitrogen mustard, used as a last-resort chemotherapy agent for lung cancer, affected patients' activities of daily living (ADLs). The scale runs from 0 to 100 and requires the clinician to rank a patient from 0 (dead) to 100 (normal; no complaints; no evidence of disease).

Despite its novelty, the Karnofsky scale was not regularly cited in published material until the late 1970s, when it emerged in cancer research due to advances in both chemotherapy and palliation (Timmermann 2013). In the 1970s chemotherapy became an established treatment for blood cancers such as leukemia and lymphoma. Shortly thereafter researchers started to apply chemotherapy to solid tumors in adults. Although chemotherapy did sometimes reduce the symptoms of solid tumor cancer, it rarely prolonged life. Chemotherapy in these cases served as a form of palliation.

The term "palliative care" was coined by Balfour Mount in 1974 following his observation of Cicely Saunder's work with the hospice movement in the United Kingdom (Loscalzo 2008). Palliative care, like hospice, focuses on the care of the whole person, including inner, spiritual life and quality of life. In the context of using chemotherapy as palliation, progress could not be measured by a lengthened life, that is, a mortality outcome. Some other form of assessment was needed. The Karnofsky scale, whose previous use had been limited, was now ready to hand, and in the 1970s parlance it qualified as a quality of life measure.

2.1.2. Emergence of the "Autonomy" Model in Medical Ethics

In his history of the Karnofsky scale, Timmermann (2013) discusses how concerns over *who* should report on quality of life preoccupied publications in the 1980s. Should clinicians report on the quality of life of their patients? Should caregivers or parents report on the quality of life of their dependents? Or should patients report on their own quality of life? Although a physician-reported scale such as Karnofsky's was unquestioned in the late 1940s, by the 1980s the medical landscape had changed. By the 1980s physicians were no longer viewed as wholly trustworthy surrogates for patients, and patients themselves were more informed and autonomous (Timmermans and Berg 2003). As Ruth Faden and Tom Beauchamp (1986) discuss in *A History and Theory of Informed Consent*, this change began in the late 1950s with the legal introduction of informed consent, an increased ethical interest in decisional authority and the doctor-patient relationship, as well as highly publicized abuses of research subjects in the United States (see also Rothman 1992).

Prior to this shift in culture, clinicians in the United States tended to operate according to a beneficence model of disclosure and consent. This model, which is oriented toward patient trust and physician obligations to provide medical benefit, imbues clinicians with moral authority and justifies them as the primary decision-makers. But from the late 1950s an autonomy model, oriented toward disclosure, consent, and patients' right to make decisions for themselves, gradually took hold. This change in climate has important consequences for who is considered a legitimate reporter of quality of life, and opened up a social, institutional, and political role for quality of life measures that previously would not have been relevant.

This "new medical ethics," as Faden and Beauchap (1986) refer to it, caught on institutionally and with it the adoption of patient-focused documents by influential organizations and bodies. For instance, in 1972, the American Hospital Association adopted the Patient's Bill of Rights, which gave patients the right to complete and current information regarding their diagnosis, treatment, and prognosis, and the right to refuse treatment. Moreover, this bill, for the first time, required doctors to incorporate patients into the decision-making process and gave to patients the right to make the final decision regarding their care. In 1982 the American Medical Association's Judicial Council recognized informed consent as a social policy that "does not accept the paternalistic view that the physician may remain silent because divulgence might prompt the patient to forego needed therapy" (Faden and Beauchamp 1986, p. 96).

Given this new patient-centered focus, it is not surprising that physician-reported measures such as the Karnofsky scale came under scrutiny. Measures that allow patients to report their own perspectives are a more natural fit for "patient centered" claims than are similar instruments whose reports about patients come from clinicians' or caregivers' perspectives. The emphasis on involving patients in reporting quality of life has only increased as it becomes clearer that family members, caregivers, and clinicians often underestimate quality of life. Moreover, they do so over diverse cultures and medical conditions (Crocker et al. 2015).

2.1.3.   Emergence of Patient-Reported Measures

If the 1970s saw the Karnofsky scale as a "quality of life measure," in the 1980s it began its life as a "patient-reported quality of life measure." In fact, being patient-reported has, over time, become a more important aspect of such measures than the content of what they measure. Since the FDA's 2009 publication *Guidance for Industry Patient-Reported Outcomes Measures: Use in Medical Product Development to Support Labeling Claims*, "patient-reported outcome measures" (PROMs) have become a popular way to refer to these instruments. Moreover, their use in health policy, journal publications, and funding applications reveals the contemporary preoccupation with them as vehicles for delivering patient-centered care.

Take for instance, the English National Health Service (NHS). In 2008 Lord Darzi presented to Parliament his review of the NHS in *High Quality Care for All*. This report envisioned an NHS for the 21st century that gave patients and the public more information, choice, and control. PROMs, which Darzi introduced as providing information about the success of treatment from the patients' point of view, were part of this vision, allowing patients themselves a voice in determining effectiveness and quality of care. In 2010 Nancy Devlin and John Appleby published with the King's Fund *Getting the Most Out of PROMs: Putting Health Outcomes at the Heart of NHS Decision-Making*. It begins with the following quotation from Donald Berwick, an American clinician, former administrator, for the Centers for Medicare and Medicaid Services, and importantly, an outspoken advocate for patient-centered care:

> The ultimate measure by which to judge the quality of a medical effort is whether it helps patients (and their families) as they see it. Anything done in health care that does not help a patient or family is, by definition, waste, whether or not the professions and their associations traditionally hallow it. (Devlin and Appleby 2010, 1, citing Berwick 1997)

Moreover, in 2013, Nick Black wrote in *British Medical Journal* that PROMs could help transform healthcare by driving changes in how it is organized and delivered, namely by giving a voice to patients' own views on their health and healthcare.

In the United States, the Centers for Medicare and Medicaid Services have employed PROMs in their Health Outcomes Survey since 1998. But PROMs came into their own in the United States in 2010 with the creation of the Patient-Centered Outcomes Research Institute (PCORI), which is funded through the Patient Protection and Affordable Care Act. PCORI's mandate is to improve the quality and relevance of evidence for patients and clinicians. It does this by funding comparative effectiveness research and focusing on outcomes important to patients. In fact, PCORI is the largest public research funder focusing primarily on comparative effectiveness research. In 2010, emphasizing the role of PROMs in comparative effectiveness research, Albert Wu and colleagues wrote in *Health Affairs* that with the creation of PCORI, "comparative effectiveness research has been renamed 'patient-centered outcomes research,' underscoring the goal of person-centered medicine" (2010, 1863). To be sure, not all of the research funded by PCORI involves PROMs, but much of it does.

Furthermore, in Denmark since 2014 there has been a push to use these measures to improve patient care and quality of care. An initiative called Program PRO (Patient-Reported Outcomes) was conducted by the Danish patient associations in collaboration with the independent nonprofit TryGonden (Egholm et al. 2023). Program PRO's goal is to improve patient involvement in the application of PROs. As a result, guidelines were developed for how patients can be involved in the planning, implementation, and sustainability of using PRO information to improve health and quality of care. For Danish healthcare, PRO data is seen as "a tool for individualizing care and making the patient an active co-partner" (Egholm et al. 2023,

104755) The use and clinical incorporation of PRO data is ongoing in Denmark.

2.2. Patient-Centered Measures? Three Concerns

Roughly speaking, prior to the publication of the FDA's *Guidance for Industry*, literature on quality of life measures tended to focus on defining these instruments in terms of their content, that is, in terms of the dimensions appropriate for inclusion in the instruments. To this end, it was common for articles to begin by distinguishing instruments by the constructs they aimed to measure: quality of life, health-related quality of life, and, possibly, health status measures (see, e.g., Guyatt et al. 1993). Increasingly—and particularly after the publication of *Guidance for Industry*—the focus is less on what these measures *are* than on what they *do*. Instead of defining a specific construct, it is now common for journal articles to present these instruments as measures that "capture patients' perspectives" (Wiering et al. 2017) or "ascertain patients' views" (Black 2013). This change in emphasis makes sense given my discussion above regarding the role they play as vehicles of patient-centered care. Yet, at the same time these instruments have been defined in terms of their ability to capture patients' perspectives, there has been significant space in high-impact journals given over to questions about whether these measures genuinely capture them. As researchers came to think of these instruments as significant for their promise to convey patients' perspectives, they also came to question their ability to do so. In what follows, I discuss three different concerns, having to do with patient input, patient individuality, and inclusivity.

2.2.1. Problematizing Patient Involvement

As early as 1997 Alain Leplège and Sonia Hunt published "The Problem of Quality of Life in Medicine" in the *Journal of the American Medical Association*. They write,

> The idea that the patients' perspective has equal validity to that of the clinician when it comes to evaluating outcomes or monitoring the effects of disease and treatment has a great deal of legitimacy and should not

be abandoned. The argument that it is the patients who are replying to questions designed by experts is not sufficient to claim that the scores calculated from these responses reflect the patients' viewpoint. (50)

Leplège and Hunt's worry is one about a lack of patient involvement and input into questionnaire development. It focuses on ensuring that patient concerns and priorities are represented in the content of these measures. I suggest their concern points toward the importance of prioritizing patient involvement when making claims of patient-centeredness.

2.2.2. Problematizing Patient Individuality

In a 2001 piece in the *British Medical Journal* Alison Carr and Irene Higginson published "Are Quality of Life Measures Patient Centered?" They argue that many of these instruments are not patient centered because standardized measuring instruments cannot cover domains and questions important to individual patients. I will treat Carr and Higginson's criticism as targeting the "nomothetic" nature of standardized quality of life and patient-reported outcome measures. "Nomothetic" is a term of art used both in philosophy and in psychology. It refers broadly to the tendency to generalize across individuals. In psychology it refers specifically to the use of statistics to describe characteristics of populations. Carr and Higginson are worried that "nomothetic" or standardized measures are *too* general to capture the nuance of individual patients. Of particular concern, the questions and possible weightings employed in any single measure may not adequately apply to all of the patients the instrument aims to hear from. For instance, leisure activities may not be important to the quality of life of some patients, while available parking at the local hospital may be very important. Carr and Higginson's concern suggests that patient-centeredness requires us to recognize the individual nature of quality of life.

2.2.3. Problematizing Patient Inclusivity

Carolyn Schwartz and Bruce Rapkin have a third concern. In 2004 they published two complementary articles in *Health and Quality of Life Outcomes* (Schwartz and Rapkin 2004; Rapkin and Schwartz 2004). In these articles they worry about the way standard psychometric models, such as classical test theory (CTT), dismiss some answers to quality of life questions as error.[2] As I discussed in Chapter 1, CTT turns on a simple model where an observed score (O) is equal to a person's true score (T) plus random error (E), thus $O = T + E$. When using CTT the value of the true score is taken to be a theoretically unknown value that is assumed to be constant, and the observed score is assumed to be a random variable that produces a bell-shaped curve around the true score. The error score is taken to have an expectation value of zero. The idea is that as the number of questionnaire administrations increases, the random errors will tend to cancel one another out; thus the mean of the observations is taken as an estimate of the true score (McClimans et al. 2017).

Schwartz and Rapkin take issue with CTT because, they argue, unlike measures of math ability, reading ability, or performance, quality of life measures should not be understood as having a constant "true score." On the contrary, they argue, answering questions about quality of life involves an appraisal, which on their view is a cognitive process involving, for example, parameters such as a frame of reference and the use of standards of comparison. This process, which can differ across cultures, personalities, situations, and time, affects how patients understand and respond to questions about their quality of life. Essentially, depending on respondents' appraisal process, they may understand and respond to questions differently than researchers intended and differently from other respondents. Nonetheless, according to Schwartz and Rapkin, the differential effects of the appraisal process should not be considered "error"; rather they argue that appraisal is part of the phenomena of quality of life. As they put this point, "The individual's particular vantage point is not arbitrary; it is intrinsic to rating of QOL" (Schwartz and Rapkin 2004).

According to Schwartz and Rapkin, the CTT model is misleading when applied to quality of life instruments. We should not expect a constant true score on a given quality of life measure, but rather what they call a "contingent true score." The contingent true score is the true score contingent upon the appraisal process used. I will discuss the appraisal model, appraisal measures, and the idea of a contingent true score at more length in Chapters 4 and 5. For my purposes here, I will treat Schwartz and Rapkin's concern in these articles as highlighting the importance of minority responses to quality of life questions. I suggest their concern points us toward the importance of inclusivity in patient-centeredness.

2.3. Responses from the Field

The three concerns above illustrate different ways in which quality of life and patient-reported instruments may fall short of being patient centered: they may lack patient input, fail to recognize patient individuality, and fail to be inclusive. These concerns are taken seriously in the literature, in policy, and with funding agencies. It is important to underline this point with specific examples because taking these concerns seriously has significant and yet philosophically counterintuitive consequences that might otherwise be easy to dismiss. There is an obvious tension between the need for a measure, which pulls in the direction of standardization, and the recognition of patient perspectives, which pulls in the direction of the individual. Unless we are clear about the criticisms and the field's response to them, it may be tempting to downplay the value of patient-centeredness and rely on standard, existing theories—theories such as subjective well-being and the capabilities approach, which I discuss in the next section—to account for these measures. Thus, in what follows I provide examples of responses to the criticisms of patient involvement, individuality, and inclusion.

2.3.1. Prioritizing Patient Involvement

In 2009 the FDA and the International Society for Pharmacoeconomics and Outcomes Research (ISPOR) both published guidelines for PROMs in the evaluation of medical products. Both sets of guidelines emphasize the importance of evidence of content validity in evaluating a PROM. Content validity evaluates how well a measuring instrument represents a sample of the construct under investigation (VandenBos 2015). These guidelines were considered revolutionary because they suggested the source of this content validity should be qualitative studies of people who have experience of the disease, illness, or disability being measured. These guidelines are a response to criticisms such as Leplège and Hunt's above: unless patients are involved in the development of a PROM, these instruments cannot claim to be representative of their perspectives (FDA 2009; Rothman et al. 2009). In tying patient involvement to issues of validity, the FDA and ISPOR underscore the integral importance of patient perspectives to developing PROMs.

2.3.2. Individualized Measures of Quality of Life

Carr and Higginson's (2001) concern that patient-centeredness requires us to recognize the individual nature of quality of life has a history that goes back to the 1990s with the creation of individualized quality of life measures, for instance, the Schedule for the Evaluation of Individual Quality of Life (SEIQoL) (O'Boyle et al. 1993) and the Patient Generated Index (PGI) (Ruta et al. 1994). I discussed these measures briefly in the introduction. These measures were developed to provide an alternative to nomothetic measures of quality of life, which critics took to exclude patients' subjective point of view. In John Browne et al.'s 1997 article "Conceptual Approaches to the Assessment of Quality of Life," the authors, clearly skeptical of nomothetic measures, state that the validity of these measures "stands and falls on the assumption that a consensus about what constitutes a good or poor quality of life exists" (738). Yet, they argue, this assumption is not empirically true. When patients are asked about what is important to them, large differences emerge in terms of domains of importance, how the domains are defined, and what the domains mean. For example, health is not always chosen by those in ill health, and when it is chosen, it can mean very different things to different people. In raising these concerns, the researchers imply that such differences are important and should be accounted for in quality of life measurement.

In order to redress the problems with nomothetic measures, individualized measures such as the SEIQoL and PGI ask patients to nominate the areas of their life that are most important to good quality and then individually weigh each dimension according to their own values. It is only with these measures, proponents argue, that we can ensure patients' perspectives are truly heard. The use of individualized measures is an important part of quality of life and PROMs research, particularly in extending the use of these measures into the clinical setting (McHorney and Tarlow 1995; Tang et al. 2014). Nonetheless, they have also been used in observational studies and feasibility studies and as a method for generating domains of interest for use in new measures (Patel et al. 2003; Nancy Mayo, pers. comm. March 2018). Nonetheless, some have expressed doubt about their ability to be used in clinical trials due to the time and cognitive requirements needed to complete them and their lack of generalizability (Patel et al. 2003). Although individualized measures are still used, their use is not ubiquitous given some of these limitations; rather, they are used in partnership with nomothetic measures or in specialized contexts.

2.3.3. Being Inclusive of Patient Perspectives

On my reading of the recent history of quality of life and PROMs, I understand Schwartz and Rapkin's (2004; Rapkin and Schwartz 2004) appraisal model as including some of the concerns embodied by proponents of individualized quality of life (such as Carr and Higginson 2001) while extending their applicability more widely. Although their orientation is different, it's possible to see Schwartz and Rapkin's criticism of CTT and the development of the appraisal model and subsequent appraisal measures as an answer to those who would argue that we need to retain standardized measures for use in, for example, clinical trials, while also maintaining a high bar for the inclusion of patient perspectives.

Schwartz and Rapkin's (2004; Rapkin and Schwartz 2004) appraisal model was developed in response to the quality of life literature on response shift. Response shift was introduced by Sprangers and Schwartz in 1999 to articulate the accommodations that many patients make to their illness. They define response shift as a change in the self-evaluation of a target construct as a result of (1) a change in the respondents' internal standards of measurement, (2) a change in the respondents' values or (3) a redefinition of the target construct (Sprangers and Schwartz 1999). The phenomenon of response shift is similar in some ways to what philosophers refer to as adaptive preference. I discuss adaptive preferences a bit more toward the end of this chapter when I talk about the capability approach to measuring well-being.

Sprangers and Schwartz argue that response shift can explain counterintuitive findings in the literature; for instance, patients with a life-threatening disease report stable quality of life, people with severe chronic illness report a level of quality of life neither inferior to nor better than less severely ill patients or healthy people, and response shift has been related to the so-called "disability paradox" (McClimans et al. 2012). Although these counterintuitive findings are traditionally treated as measurement error, the literature on response shift has tried to correct this treatment, arguing that these findings represent important and relevant information about patient perspectives on quality of life. Yet as a theoretical construct, response shift had limited success in the face of traditional psychometric models such as CTT. The introduction of the appraisal model and subsequent appraisal measures, however, provide a way of measuring response shift, and thus, in my view, provide more potential for integrating an inclusive range of patient perspectives into quality of life research.

The development of appraisal measures (Rapkin et al. 2017, 2018) was funded by PCORI for a little over $1 million. You will recall PCORI funds research on comparative effectiveness research. Clinical trials play an important role in comparative effectiveness research, and thus it is reasonable to expect that measures of response shift will have a role in clinical trials, bringing a more inclusive array of patient perspectives to this area of research. Once again, I will have more to say about response shift and the appraisal model in Chapters 4 and 5. For now I simply want to point out that Schwartz and Rapkin's (2004; Rapkin and Schwartz 2004) work on appraisal embodies some of the ethical concerns of inclusion that we saw at the heart of the movement for individualized quality of life while possibly extending their applicability to clinical trials. This is important since, as I discussed above, individualized quality of life measures themselves are limited in terms of practical applications due to time and cognitive requirements, as well as questions about generalizability.

2.4. Toward a Theory of Patient-Centered Measurement

Health researchers, major medical journals, policy bodies, and funding agencies are concerned that quality of life measures and PROMs are patient centered. Philosophy can serve a practical end in this field by articulating a vision of patient-centeredness that respects the concerns researchers raise about quality of life and PROMs, while also linking to relevant literature in medical ethics and disability studies. To do this, I suggest we consider quality of life and PROMs as a distinct category of measuring instrument. I refer to these instruments as *patient-centered* measures. My discussion above serves as the foundation for two requirements of patient-centeredness:

1. Prioritize patient involvement
2. Be inclusive of patient perspectives

Patients should be involved in the development of patient-centered measures, and these measures should be inclusive of a range of respondent perspectives. The first requirement speaks to Leplège and Hunt's (1997) concern about patient involvement in the development of PROMs, but also that of Trujols and Portella (2013), who write that PROMs need to reflect patients' views and concerns. It is also consistent with FDA and ISPOR guidance, which I discuss at more length in the next chapter. It is not enough to have patients report on their quality of life or physical functioning when the questions asked are based on what clinicians and researchers think matter: patient-centeredness requires patients' concerns and priorities be represented in the measure's content. Moreover, patient-centered measures should be inclusive of a range of respondent answers that reflect different values, interests, and understandings. This second requirement speaks to Rapkin and Schwartz's (2004; Schwartz and Rapkin 2004) concern that differences in respondent understandings of, for example, what quality of life is do not necessarily indicate measurement error. It also speaks to interests articulated by the individualized quality of life movement, whose advocates argue against a one-sized-fits-all approach to these measures. I discuss inclusion in patient-centered measures at more length in Chapter 4.

The sentiment embodied in my two requirements for patient-centeredness echo the "new medical ethics," where patient autonomy overshadows beneficence and best interests. This ethic influenced discussions in quality of life and PROMs research regarding who should report on the quality of life of patients. It also helped to create a need for patient representation in comparative effectiveness research and research on quality of care. But if health journals, health policies, and funding agencies recognize the importance of making quality of life and patient-reported instruments patient centered, philosophical approaches have tended to overlook this point. Instead, philosophical approaches to quality of life measures have often associated them with measures of well-being. In this section I discuss two examples and argue that neither captures what's at stake in *patient-centered* measures. First, I take up measures of subjective well-being, and then I turn to measures of the capability approach to quality of life.

2.4.1. Subjective Well-Being

Ed Deiner was an American psychologist who developed the contemporary model for well-being in 1984. This influential model measures well-being, or "happiness," along three dimensions: life satisfaction and positive and negative affect. Patient-centered measures are sometimes associated with measures of subjective well-being—and indeed there are similarities. Erik Angner (2011), for instance, appropriates patient-centered measures in mental health and gerontology for subjective well-being. Yet, while there are similarities between patient-centered measures and measures of subjective well-being—they are first-person reported, they are designed most often as questionnaires, they can share dimensions of interest—they are different in at least two important ways. First, while measures of subjective well-being are measured along three standardized dimensions, patient-centered measures are measured along a variety of non-standardized dimensions. Second, their purpose is different. Measures of subjective well-being are geared toward improving society; patient-centered measures are geared toward capturing patients' perspectives.

As I discussed in the previous chapter, we don't have settled answers to questions about the meaning of constructs such as quality of life with urinary incontinence or subjective functioning after a spinal cord injury (and as I'll discuss further in Chapter 4, this is a feature, not a glitch). The upshot is that different patient-centered measures can conceptualize the same construct differently. For instance, the International Consultation on Incontinence (ICIQ-SF) and the Incontinence Impact Questionnaire-7 (IIQ-7) are both used to diagnose individuals with urinary incontinence and assess the impact of dysfunction on patient quality of life (Skorupska et al. 2021). But the ICIQ-SF evaluates frequency, severity, and impact of urinary incontinence on quality of life, while the IIQ-7 focuses on psychosocial impact of urinary incontinence on women. And these are not the only urinary incontinence-specific quality of life measures! There are others like the Urinary Distress Inventory-7, which also aims to measure the same construct with yet a third emphasis.

Measures of subjective well-being, however, are not as diverse. Indeed, one of Deiner's major contributions to the field of psychology was to standardize the definition of subjective well-being and streamline its measurement (Ng et al. 2021). Subjective well-being refers to the degree to which people feel their life is going well. It is measured via life satisfaction. Life satisfaction is measured on three dimensions: a cognitive component and positive and negative affect; affects are feeling states such as emotion and mood (Deiner et al. 1999). Positive affect assesses the extent to which an individual subjectively experiences positive moods such as joy, and negative affect assesses the experience of negative emotions and poor self-concept, such as anger, guilt, and nervousness.

While some patient-centered measures include questions about positive and negative affect, they also regularly include a wide variety of other dimensions. Take for instance, the European Organization for Research and Treatment of Cancer Quality of Life Questionnaire (EORTC QLQ-C30). This instrument has two global health status questions; five different functional scales (e.g., role functioning and social functioning); and nine symptom scales (e.g., fatigue and diarrhea) (EORTC 2002). This instrument does not look like a measure of subjective well-being. The Breast-Q, a patient-centered measure for cosmetic and reconstructive breast surgery, however, more closely resembles a measure of subjective well-being because it focuses on satisfaction and affect. It includes questions about satisfaction with breasts, overall outcome, and process of care, as well as questions about psychosocial, physical, and sexual well-being (Pusic et al. 2009). The Spitzer Quality of Life Index (SQLI), yet again, however, includes questions that cover activities of daily living, health, support of family and friends, and outlook (Spitzer et al. 1981). Like the EORTC QLQ-C30, the SQLI does not resemble subjective well-being.

While patient-centered measures often include questions about positive and negative affect and, less often, questions about satisfaction, they usually include other dimensions. This diversity makes sense considering the unsettled nature of these constructs and the unrestricted way that these measures are usually developed, that is, from clinicians and researcher interests and observations or, more recently, from patients' experiences. The diversity of dimensions found in patient-centered measures raises questions about their similarity to measures of subjective well-being. This skepticism is strengthened when we turn to the history of these measures to understand better their respective purposes.

The most important difference in the historical development of these measures rests in the motivation that led to the development of patient-centered measures. Recall from my earlier discussion that patient-centered measures developed out of a desire to capture *patients'* (not clinicians') points of view. Put differently, patient-centered measures were influenced by a movement in medical ethics that turned away from beneficence to patient autonomy. Yet when Angner (2011) discusses the motivation that led to the development of measures of subjective well-being, he argues for beneficence. In fact, Angner argues that the history of measures of subjective well-being conforms to the history of social and behavioral measurement explored in Theodore Porter's *Trust in Numbers*. Both developed out of an impetus to improve society. Porter (1995) clarifies this moral impulse. He writes:

Much, probably most, statistical study of human populations has aimed to improve the condition of working people, children, beggars, criminals, women or racial and ethnic minorities. The writings, especially private ones, of early social statisticians and pioneers of the social survey exude benevolence and goodwill. . . . Middle class philanthropists and social workers used statistics to learn about kinds of people whom they did not know, and often did not care to know, as persons. Counting was not impeded, but encouraged, by their alienness, for averages must always appear less meaningful when drawn from a population of strong and interesting personalities. *A method of study that ignored individuality seemed right* for the lower classes. (77, italics mine)

In this passage Porter describes what I refer to as a benevolence model of moral impulse. On the benevolence model, actions are taken in the best interests of others. When applied to measurement (as opposed to, for instance, medicine) best interests are geared toward populations, not individuals. Thus, the benevolence model focuses on what is good for a population independent of individual perspectives on this good. Angner (2011) echoes this benevolence model in his discussion of what drove, and continues to drive, research in subjective well-being. He emphasizes the role benevolence plays in public and social policy. For instance, he discusses the need for policymakers to understand the causal antecedents that lead to a happy marriage, so that they can promote happy marriages in public policy. In this context, policymakers are not interested in the unique qualities of individual happy marriages or learning about the intricacies of how a happy marriage varies from couple to couple and over time. Rather, Angner's policymakers, similar to the researchers Porter describes, are interested in applying general causal principles to the entire population to improve the likelihood of a generic happy marriage. Accordingly, they tend to treat individual perspectives on marriage as noise.

As for patient-centered measures, policy is also one of the contexts in which they are used, and one of these policy purposes is to improve the quality of healthcare. But as I discussed above, the main reason these measures are included in healthcare quality improvement research is to signal a commitment to patient-centered care. The Institute of Medicine includes patient-centered care as one of six domains of healthcare quality. Patient-centered care is defined in *Crossing the Quality Chasm* (2001) as "providing care that is respectful of and responsive to *individual patient* preferences, needs, and values and ensuring that patient values guide all clinical decisions" (6, italics mine). Notice the emphasis on the individual. In health policy, patient-centered measurement aims to contribute to better-quality healthcare, but the moral impulse it epitomizes is best characterized by what I call an autonomy model of moral impulse, not a benevolence model. An autonomy model recognizes the importance of individual perspectives both because first-person accounts are valuable and because individual differences matter. How the autonomy model should be applied to patient-centered measures is what this book is about, but as an instance of the benevolence model, subjective well-being is not the appropriate theoretical framework for patient-centered measurement.

2.4.2. Capability Approach to Quality of Life

The capability approach to quality of life is often seen as a philosophical model for quality of life measures and PROMs. Prominent bioethicists as well as health researchers have made this connection (e.g., Brock 1993; Verkerk et al. 2001; van Loon et al. 2018). Indeed, some quality of life measures and PROMs do resemble the capability approach. But my argument here is that as *patient-centered* measures, as measures that aim for patient prioritization and inclusion, the capability approach is the wrong approach. To understand why, we need to dig a bit into the capability approach and what motivated its development.

In 1979 the Indian economist and philosopher Amartya Sen delivered a critique of earlier understandings of how well-being might be measured in society in his Tanner Lecture on Human Value "Equality of What" (Sen 1979). In this lecture he criticized three approaches to equality as a measure of well-being. One comes from the American philosopher John Rawls, who related well-being to a person's access to "primary goods"; the other two come from utilitarianism and welfare economics, which in different ways relate well-being to "utility." The capability approach to quality of life—an objective list theory of well-being—emerged out of Sen's lecture (Sen 1979, 218–220). Before I discuss the capability approach and objective list theories, let's look at Sen's criticisms of primary goods and utility as measures of well-being.

Consider first Sen's critique of primary goods. According to Rawls ([1971] 1999, 54–55), primary goods help articulate what resources individuals need to be reasonable and rational citizens. For instance, individuals should have the capacity to develop and pursue their own conception of what is a good quality of life. But this capacity is contingent on access to certain resources, resources such as freedom of movement, free to choose from a wide range of occupations, income, wealth, and so on. These resources are what Rawls refers to as "primary goods." For Rawls, a just society is one that maximizes these primary goods across citizens. Yet Sen and others (Nagel 1973; Schwartz 1973) have argued that the usefulness of primary goods differs depending on both the capacities individuals begin with and what they value. Sen is particularly concerned with how human diversity affects our need for primary goods. People with disabilities or chronic illness, or even pregnant women, may need more primary goods than others to develop and pursue what they take to be a good quality of life. For instance, if I use a wheelchair and I want to pursue a public education, then I will probably need use of a wheelchair-accessible vehicle. These vehicles are often more expensive than non-accessible vehicles, and thus I will require more resources—primary goods—in the form of income or wealth to pursue a public education than someone who does not use a wheelchair.

Now consider Sen's critique of utility as a measure of well-being. Utility construes pleasure, satisfaction, or happiness as well-being. Yet some people are hard to please and others are easy. Should those who need more from life to be happy get more resources than those who need less? And what about those who adapt to their circumstances? When our circumstances constrict our options and we learn to be happy with less, is this a problem? Should a person with a disability who, for instance, claims to adapt happily to life without hearing or certain kinds of mobility be taken at face value? This latter example speaks to the problem of adaptive preferences. To be sure, most of us have the experience of adapting preferences to our circumstances. As a child I wanted a round house, and I continued to want one until I realized the expense of architecturally designed homes. In the end, I was happy to get a mortgage that put a roof over my head no matter the shape of it. But I also grew up without regular access to hot water or a telephone. But I got used to these conditions too and came to think of my bracing cold-water hair wash as a surefire way of waking up quickly in the morning. If adapting to the reality of the property market is sensible, what about adapting to these other conditions? When is preference adaptation problematic, and when it is pragmatic?[3]

Sen's capability approach aims to resolve this question about adaptive preferences as well as the problem of diverse needs by focusing not on a set of defined resources (primary goods) to which we should have access *or* what circumstances people prefer, but rather what capacities people have. The idea is that justice requires the state to ensure that people have a set of basic capacities. If people have these basic capacities, then they can use them to develop a good-quality life as they see fit. But if these capacities are missing, then the idea is that individual choices aren't properly free. Some of the capacities that have been included in this approach are these: being able to live to the end of a human life of normal length, being able to have good health, and having adequate nutrition, adequate shelter, opportunities for sexual satisfaction and choice in reproduction, and mobility (Nussbaum 2000). The capability approach is often called an "objective list" theory of well-being because it assumes that the capacities required to develop a good-quality life benefit everyone independent of whether individuals in fact endorse them. I may be asexual and thus not personally appreciate opportunities for sexual satisfaction. Nonetheless, objective list theories hold that having such opportunities is good for me; indeed, having these opportunities makes my choices not to engage in sex free choices.

The capability approach holds fixed the kinds of activities in which citizens should be able to partake, and the kinds of people citizens should be free to become instead of the resources or utility needed to achieve them (Robeyns and Byskov 2020). At the core of the capability approach are two special concepts that I'll explain momentarily: "functionings" and "capabilities." Capabilities refer to the opportunities people have even if they choose not to fulfill them. For instance, one can have the capacity for sexual satisfaction and yet not partake in it; for instance, one might be asexual. Functionings, on the other hand, refer to personal achievements. They include achievements such as getting into and out of a bath on one's own, walking to the shops, participating in leisure activities, or socializing with friends.

Most measures employing the capability approach track respondents' functionings, that is, their achievements. Indeed, this is how Dan Brock (1993) interpreted quality of life measures and PROMs when he claimed them for the capability approach in his article "Quality of Life Measures in Health Care and Medical Ethics." Brock (1993) treated the individual dimensions of the Sickness Impact Profile (SIP), Quality of Life Index (QLI), and Health Status Index—dimensions such as "Recreation and Pastimes" and "Body Care and Movement"—as functionings. For Brock, these functionings refer to centrally important activities that, when missing from respondents' lives, limit their choices or opportunities in creating and pursuing different life plans. The questions within each of these dimensions thus assess the impact of disease or illness on quality of life by gathering information about how well respondents are able to perform the requisite functioning. Take the SIP as an example. It asks for responses to questions such as "I am going out for entertainment less" or "I do not bathe myself at all but am bathed by someone else." These questions relate to functionings within the dimensions of "Recreation and Pastimes" and "Body Care and Movement," respectively. Respondents who achieve less, for example, go out less, have someone else bathe them, are measured as having a less good life.

The capability approach as applied to quality of life measures and PROMs is not meant to evaluate a particular life plan. It doesn't intend to speak to the value of, for instance, having a disability or not having one, being healthy or having a chronic illness. Rather it is meant to assess the extent to which a cohort of patients is sufficiently free to choose a life plan, whether their functionings permit a sufficient level of freedom. The idea is that a biological condition, say, deafness or fibromyalgia, doesn't, on its own, make quality of life poor. Rather, it's the loss of achievement that may accompany deafness or fibromyalgia, for instance, deficits in oral communication or mobility, that decreases quality of life.[4] Moreover, respondents who report a loss of functioning are measured as having a lower quality of life even if they report subjectively having a high quality of life. By holding the functionings as a constant threshold of a good quality of life, measures that employ the capability approach attempt to redress the question of problematic adaptive preferences.

Brock is not the only person to recognize the similarity between some quality of life measures and PROMs and the capabilities approach; others have also made this connection (e.g., Verkerk et al. 2001; van Loon et al. 2018). And they are correct that there are similarities: like the capability approach, many of these measures treat the answers to questions within each dimension as affecting the measurement score independent of what respondents might otherwise report about the quality of their lives. Moreover, as I discussed above when considering individualized quality of life, nomothetic or standardized instruments assume that the same dimensions are important to everyone; that is, the same primary functionings denote valuable opportunities for all. Despite these similarities, *patient-centered* measures should not be understood as instantiations of the capability approach.

As I discussed above, one motivation behind Sen's development of the capabilities approach is to correct for adaptive preferences. The capability approach was developed in large part to stand fast in the face of adaptive preferences and hold fixed certain capabilities for everyone. Yet as I discussed earlier in this chapter, in the health literature, adaptive preferences—usually referred to as response shifts—are increasingly understood as representing important and relevant information about patient perspectives on patient-centered constructs like quality of life. Indeed, some medical specialties, such as rehabilitation or palliative care, aim to create response shifts in their patient populations (Barclay-Goddard et al. 2009). Doing so is considered an achievement of quality of life, not a preference for something suboptimal. Moreover, literature on transformative epistemic experiences (Paul 2014) suggests that we cannot assign a value to experiences to which we do not have epistemic assess. Many disability cases, including those of deaf individuals who consider cochlear implantation, are like this. In cases such as these, we need to do more than assume we know in advance what functionings, such as oral communication, are valuable to a good-quality life. What "more" do we need to do? We need to practice epistemic humility, which I discussed in Chapter 1. We need to be open to being wrong about what we think makes for a good-quality life.

What we might call a "first person" perspective in measurement (which characterizes patient-centered measures) is morally different from the "third person" perspective that motivates the capability approach. Inclusive patient-centered instruments must embody the ability to learn from patients. Whether through appraisal measures or some other mechanism, inclusive instruments need to be sensitive to new ways in which a life can have quality. When applied to healthcare, the capabilities approach tends to assume that we already know the functionings required for a good-quality life. This is not an adequate theory for instruments shaped and popularized by contemporary medical ethics.

2.5. Conclusion

The historical development of quality of life instruments and patient-reported measures, which I call patient-centered measures, situates them at the vertex of two very different trends in medicine: patient-centered care and standardization. The historical sketch that I provide in this chapter illustrates how these instruments have evolved to meet the contingencies of the previous eighty years. The Karnofsky Performance Scale began life as a measure of patients' burden on a society whose aim was to better measure the progress of highly toxic chemotherapy agents. The scale was physician reported, and, rather than concern itself with patient perspectives, it seems to have been part of the culture that Siddhartha Mukerjee (2010) refers to as the "smiling oncologist"—the doctor who genially prescribes poisons to patients in the hopes of a cure. Yet from the beginnings of the Karnofsky scale we find ourselves decades later with a collection of measures caught up in the "new medical ethic" focused on capturing patients' perspectives.

Without an understanding of the history of quality of life measures and PROMs, it would be easy to dismiss characterizations of "capturing patients' perspective" as mere rhetoric designed to rally public support. But this interpretation is not correct. When major medical journals, policy bodies, and funding agencies put time, energy, and money into criticisms and solutions, then that concern is real. It is this concern—how to make these instruments patient centered—that separates these instruments from other, more philosophically familiar ones. I suggest two requirements for patient-centered measures:

1. Prioritize patient-centered involvement
2. Be inclusive of patient perspectives

Measures of subjective well-being and measures that embody the capability approach to quality of life are sometimes suggested as theoretical frameworks for quality of life measures and PROMs. But these theories will not do for patient-centered measures. On the one hand, patient-centered measures cannot be understood as measures of subjective well-being because they are committed to an autonomy model of patient input, not a benevolence model. On the other hand, patient-centered measures should not be taken as an example of the capability approach to quality of life. Despite the fact that nomothetic measures do roughly follow the logic of the capability approach, this logic does not allow for a sufficiently responsive instrument, and thus discriminates against the quality of life or functioning of those it does not understand. The capability approach is not inclusive.

When we accept that quality-of-life instruments and PROMs are patient-centered measures, this recognition has far-reaching consequences for how to theorize about these measures. In the next two chapters I develop an epistemic theory of patient-centered measures, first focusing on the criterion of prioritizing patient involvement and then, in Chapter 4, turning to inclusion.

PART II
AN EPISTEMIC THEORY
FOR PATIENT-CENTERED
MEASURES

3

Epistemic Dialogue

In the previous chapter I argued that patient-centered measures should be understood as distinct from measures in the social sciences to which they are sometimes compared, namely measures of subjective well-being and objective list measures. The primary reason I gave is we cannot separate the rise in popularity of patient-centered measures from their role in representing and amplifying patients' perspectives. Patient-centered measures are often used to represent the "patients' voice" in research and regulatory contexts. The nature of this representation is due to a historical context that emphasizes patient autonomy and patient expertise. I further argued that patient-centered measures are *patient centered* to the degree that they (1) prioritize patient involvement and (2) are inclusive of patient perspectives.

In this chapter I further develop the first of these criteria with the aim of laying down the foundations of an epistemic theory for patient-centered measures. Most of this development focuses on the ethical and epistemic importance of prioritizing involvement of people with disabilities, patients, and other ill persons in the development of patient-centered measures. Toward the end of the chapter, however, I develop an approach to prioritizing patient involvement that I call epistemic dialogue. Epistemic dialogue helps to foreground and take seriously marginalized testimony from the first-person perspective, but it also provides a role for secondhand perspectives, such as those of health researchers. Thus, prioritizing patient involvement in measure development does not mean acquiescing to patient points of view; rather, it means coming to understand better the constructs patient-centered measures aim to access while making the most of the expertise people with disabilities, patients, and other ill people have.

In recent decades it has become common for the host of different patient-centered measures to be framed in terms of their purpose, that is, to capture patients' perspectives, rather than in terms of the specific construct they aim to measure. This change roughly maps onto the change in nomenclature of "quality of life measures" to the somewhat awkward, yet descriptive "patient-reported outcome measures" (PROMs). Some have interpreted this change

Patient-Centered Measurement. Leah M. McClimans, Oxford University Press. © Oxford University Press 2024.
DOI: 10.1093/oso/9780197572078.003.0004

as an attempt to avoid difficult theoretical and methodological questions about measuring quality of life. Anna Alexandrova (2017, xiv) writes, "When medical researchers study the so-called patient reported outcomes (PROs) . . . they sometimes distance themselves from the term 'well-being.'" She goes on to attribute this distance to belief that patient-reported effectiveness is more tractable than well-being or because researchers are trying to "weasel out of hard questions." Although researchers in some contexts do distance themselves from quality of life as a construct of interest—and no doubt sometimes this is due to its complexity—the reasons for doing so are varied. As I discussed in the previous chapter, quality of life measures and PROMs became popular evaluative tools in large part because they dovetail with an increasingly emancipated patient population, and also because of a social, institutional, and legal context that increasingly recognizes the need to incorporate patient perspectives. From this standpoint the emphasis on patient reports is best understood as an attempt to further the patient-focused agenda. This agenda pervades healthcare, extending from the philosophically familiar context of the clinic to the less familiar context of measurement and the evaluation of care.

In the previous chapter, the policy examples I gave were largely taken from comparative effectiveness research. But patient-centered measures are also used in other areas of evaluation, perhaps most notably to support medical product-labeling claims. In the first part of this chapter, I provide a recent history of the Food and Drug Administration's (FDA) involvement with PROMs. This example is intended to illustrate how bringing patient-centered measures into the fold of medical outcomes research has had an important consequence for their methodology. In a reversal of most previous validation practices in this area, the FDA prioritizes content over construct validity. This change has philosophical implications.

Philosophers interested in the measurement of well-being have traditionally focused on "prudential" theories that offer competing accounts of well-being, meaning that they offer competing accounts of what is good for a person.[1] The questions they ask are largely concerned with what is intrinsically good for a person, meaning that questions of what well-being is are answered without reference to how well-being can bring about other good ends. Rather, well-being is considered a good in itself, a good that we desire for its own sake. The "Big Three" contenders, as Alexandrova (2017) refers to them, are hedonism, desire theories, and objective list theories. Perhaps well-being consists in the greatest balance of pleasure over pain. Or maybe it consists in satisfying my informed desires. Alternatively, well-being might consist in an objective list of items irreducible to pleasure or desires, items such as friendship, mobility, and practical reasoning, similar to the capability approach discussed in Chapter 2 (Finnis 2011; Nussbaum 2000; Griffin 1986; Sen 1984). Although, as I argued previously, patient-centered measures are not independent from questions of well-being, focusing on answers to questions of prudential value ignores the contemporary context of these measures.

In the contemporary context, patient-centered measures are increasingly framed in terms of their purpose, *not their construct*. This purpose—to capture patient perspectives, to represent the patient's voice—is part of larger agenda of patient-centered care. As I will argue, this purpose finds new purchase in the FDA's emphasis on content over construct validity. If philosophy is to be useful in the context of this methodological shift, we need a different philosophical approach. Instead of focusing on prudential theory and asking in what the target construct might consist, we should aim for an epistemic theory that focuses on people with disabilities', patients', and other ill persons' contributions to the development of the construct in question. In other words, a philosophical approach fitting contemporary patient-centered measures should focus on the process through which constructs like quality of life are developed.

3.1. FDA and PROMs

In the regulatory context the FDA has been steadily increasing patient engagement since 1988 (FDA 2020). In 2001, as part of its interest in patient engagement, the FDA heard formal presentations from the Patient-Reported Outcome Harmonization Group (PRO Harmonization Group), whose members came from the International Society for Quality of Life Research, the International Society for Pharmacoeconomics and Outcomes Research (ISPOR), the Pharmaceutical Manufacturer's Association Health Outcomes Committee, and the European Regulatory Issues on Quality of Life Assessment. The aim of the PRO Harmonization Group was to coordinate outcomes review criteria for United States and European regulatory agencies (Acquadro et al. 2003). In their presentations to the FDA these groups focused on the definition and operation of PROs, their added value in the regulatory process, PRO methodology, and the interest and demand for PRO information by decision-makers.

The PRO Harmonization Group's lobbying effort was ultimately successful. In 2009 the FDA published guidance for industry on the use of PROMs and identified their purpose: "to capture the patient's experience" (FDA 2009). The FDA could have understood their purpose differently, for instance, as quantifying health-related quality of life or providing information on adverse side-effects (as indeed some FDA officials in a 1989 study understood their potential; see Luce et al. 1989). Their chosen purpose, however, fit with the FDA's interest in expanding these instruments from measuring health-related quality of life to serving the broader goal of patient engagement.

This interest continues apace. In 2012, as part of the fifth reauthorization of the Prescription Drug User Fee Act (PDUFA), the FDA explicitly began including patient perspectives in the regulatory review process as part of its Patient-Focused Drug Development Program (PFDD) (FDA 2020; 2022). These perspectives were sought through 24 public disease-specific meetings covering conditions such as autism, Parkinson's Disease and female sexual dysfunction (FSD). One key conclusion from these meetings was that patients should be considered experts in what it is like to live with their condition(s) (FDA 2017).

In 2016, with the signing of the 21st Century Cures Act and the 2017 reauthorization of PDUFA, Congress directed the FDA to produce guidance on methods and approaches for capturing and measuring patient perspectives and experiences (FDA 2020). This set of guidances is understood by the FDA as providing fit-for-purpose tools that will allow the systematic collection of patient perspectives and experiences, thus serving as a bridge from the kind of information collected in the PFDD public meetings to standardized settings, for instance, clinical trials (FDA 2017). Between 2018 and 2023 the FDA drafted and produced four sets of PFDD guidance covering how stakeholders can collect and submit patient experience data for medical product development and regulatory decision-making. Guidances 3 and 4 cover the methods and technologies of clinical outcome assessments (COAs), which supplement the 2009 PROMs Guidance for Industry (FDA 2023). "COAs" is the general term the FDA uses to refer to instruments, such as patient-centered measures, that may be influenced by human choice, judgment, or motivation, which support evidence of treatment benefit. In addition to patient-centered measures, COAs include clinician-reported, observer-reported, and performance outcome measures.

In thinking about the evolution of patient-centered measures, it is important to recognize the historical role that institutions, policy documents, and legal frameworks play. In the case of regulation in the United States, both industry and the FDA were looking for ways to include patient perspectives in their processes. Quality of life measures eventually came to be understood as fulfilling this need. We should not be surprised, given the hermeneutic structure of coordination in measurement, that these instruments themselves were changed as a result. Measures that in the 1980s were variously characterized as health status, quality of life, and health-related quality of life came to be understood in most institutional contexts as *patient*-reported outcome measures. And with this change in nomenclature has come changes in priorities, for instance, less interest in what it means to measure quality of life, more interest in ensuring that patient views are adequately represented. As I will discuss in the next section, this change in priorities has also accompanied changes in measurement methodology.

3.2. The Rise of Content Validity

Since the 1980s, industry had been using the outcomes from quality of life measures in its applications to the FDA (Luce et al. 1989). Nonetheless, as Luce et al. (1989) found in their interviews with FDA officials, the administration at the time remained unconvinced that these measures represented genuinely new instruments. To a large degree, these doubts were well founded. Many of the instruments first dubbed "quality of life" were similar to the Karnofsky scale, that is, originally developed as something else. The Karnofsky scale, as I discussed in Chapter 2, was originally designed as a performance scale modeled on activities of daily living (ADLs). ADLs are meant to represent the adequacy of neurological and locomotor systems, not quality of life (Mayo 2015). When, almost 30 years later in 2009, the FDA recognized these measures with "Guidance for Industry Patient-Reported Outcomes Measures: Use in Medical Product Development to Support Labeling Claims," the skepticism about the term "quality of life" remained. Although the term does not feature in the text of the guidance itself, in the glossary it is defined as the following:

Quality of life: A general concept that implies an evaluation of the effect of all aspects of life on general well-being. Because this term implies the evaluation of nonhealthy-related aspects of life, and because the term generally is accepted to mean *what the patient thinks it is*, it is too general and undefined to be considered appropriate for a medical product claim. (FDA 2009, 33)

In place of quality of life, the FDA seems to prefer "health-related quality of life," which is defined as a "multidomain concept that represents the patient's general perception of the effect of illness and treatment on physical, psychological, and social aspects of life" (FDA 2009, 32). But, interestingly, as with "quality of life," "health-related quality of life" is not mentioned outside of the glossary. When it comes to specifying what PROMs measure, the FDA is vague:

In clinical trials, a PRO instrument can be used to measure the effect of a medical intervention on one or more concepts (i.e., the *thing* being measured, such as a symptom or group of symptoms, effect on a particular function or group of functions, or a group of symptoms or functions shown to measure the severity of a health conditions). (FDA 2009, 2)

Where the FDA is somewhat vague about the construct being measured, it is quite detailed about the evidence needed to support the validity of that construct. It defines content validity in this way:

Evidence from qualitative research demonstrating that the instrument measures the concept of interest including evidence that the items and domains of an instrument are appropriate and comprehensive relative to its intended measurement concept, population, and use. Testing other measurement properties will not replace or rectify problems with content validity. (FDA 2009, 31)

There are six and a half pages in the guidance discussing content validity compared to three pages that discuss "other measurement properties," that is, reliability, construct validity, and responsiveness. When determining the adequacy of an instrument, the FDA requires the following documentation on content validity:

- A literature review on the measure's concept and documentation of expert input.

- Qualitative study protocols, interview guides and summary of results for any patient focus groups, open-ended patient interviews and/or cognitive interviews.
- The origin and derivation of items with the chronology of events for item generation, modification and finalization, item tracking matrix for versions tested with patients showing the items retained and deleted, and showing evidence of saturation.
- A qualitative study summary that supports content validity for (1) item content, (2) response options, (3) recall period, and (4) scoring.
- A summary of qualitative studies demonstrating how the item pool was generated, reduced, and finalized along with specification of the type of qualitative study used and the characteristics of the study population. (FDA 2009, 36–37)

This emphasis on content validity is both unusual and telling. It's unusual because since roughly 1989 with Messick's notion of "unified validity," construct validity has been more or less king, subsuming content and criterion validity. Indeed, Messick (1980) argued that content validity isn't properly speaking even a kind of validity. Regardless, in the FDA's guidance this priority is undone: content validity leads the way, with construct validity denigrated to "Other Validity."

This reversal does not mean that the FDA has no interest in the conceptual framework of these measures—it does. But what seems to be at stake for the FDA is whether the concept has been operationalized in a way that is consistent with the views of the intended population. In a field typically dominated by quantitative research, this emphasis on qualitative work is striking. We might say that the FDA is concerned that these measures be context sensitive. It seems to be somewhat less concerned with the degree to which an instrument's items conform to a priori hypotheses regarding related concepts, or scores produced from measures with similar or diverse populations—in other words, less concerned with construct validity.

If the emphasis on content validity is unusual, it is also telling. It signals an official shift from, nominally, theory-driven measures to explicitly patient-driven ones. As I discuss in the previous chapter, the shift to patient-centered measures has been a few decades coming. But the 2009 FDA guidance signals a methodological shift from emphasizing construct validity to content validity. The significance of this shift is to move the responsibility for the content of the construct from researchers to patients.

As I discussed in Chapter 1, in Cronbach and Meehl's classic 1955 paper, construct validity is usually taken to require a theory of the construct being measured or a nomological net (nomological nets describe the relationships between the construct and other variables). Because construct validity is usually taken to be the most important validity metric, textbooks use the language of theory to describe the validation of these measures (Streiner and Norman 2007). As I also discussed in Chapter 1, in practice construct validity is usually determined by statistical correlations (CTT) or item fit (Rasch), and this practice has led to many criticisms of shoddy validation (Alexandrova and Haybron 2016; Cano and Hobart 2011). Even if in practice these instruments are not theory driven, until late in the first decade of this century, they were nominally so. The FDA's emphasis on content validity, however, changes their status from nominally theory driven to patient driven. This emphasis methodologically aligns these instruments with the FDA's patient-focused priorities; it also goes some way toward setting the persistent criticism of theory deficiency to one side.

It's important to note the FDA is not alone in making the methodological shift of prioritizing content validity. In 2009 ISPOR published the results of a task force to address good clinical research practices for the use of existing or modified PROMs (Rothman et al. 2009). These results focus on the importance of content validity and the use of qualitative research as evidence of it. In 2007, in an effort to develop a method for choosing among PROMs based on their quality, Caroline Terwee and colleagues (2007) at Vrije Universiteit developed quality criteria for health status questionnaires. Their criteria included the usual suspects: content validity, construct validity, internal consistency, responsiveness, and so on. But Terwee's team (2007) prioritized content validity as the one necessary quality threshold that all measures must meet before they can be considered for use.

Not everyone agrees with this emphasis on content validity. In her book *A Philosophy for the Science of Well-Being*, Alexandrova (2017) discusses the move to use patients to validate measures of well-being. Alexandrova's interest is in well-being measures generally speaking, and thus not limited to patient-centered measures specifically, but her discussion of what she calls "evidentiary subjectivism" uses examples from the PROMs literature. Evidentiary subjectivism refers to a position on the kind of evidence needed to validate a well-being questionnaire, in this case, reports (or behavior) from the relevant population. Alexandrova (2017, 140–41) develops two kinds of evidentiary subjectivism, conversational and behavioral. The behavioral version refers to statistical techniques used in the construct validation of patient-centered measures, while the conversational version refers to respondent self-reports. I'll focus on the conversational version, which maps onto the FDA's and ISPOR's criteria for content validity.

How do we know if a patient-centered measure asks the right questions about whatever it is trying to measure? If we ask about pain at night or fatigue walking 100 meters, how do we know whether the answers to these questions will help us to understand, say, quality of life in postoperative cancer patients, or pain in people with rheumatoid arthritis? What evidence would count in favor of a particular question being a good one? As I discussed above, the FDA, ISPOR, and others emphasize qualitative evidence from the patient population to support the item pool, item content, response options, recall period, and scoring. Alexandrova (2017, 141) refers to this kind of methodology as conversational evidential subjectivism: "Conversational evidential subjectivism: Φ should be accepted as a component of x's well-being only if φ is a self-report of a factor systematically claimed to be valued by subjects relevantly similar to x in a well-designed interview or survey." To be sure, neither in practice nor in principle is the content validity of PROMs entirely reliant on this form of evidential subjectivism. For instance, the FDA guidance is interested in respondent input, but also literature reviews and expert contributions. Moreover, as I discussed in the previous chapter, one complaint of the FDA's emphasis on content validity is that it is often ignored because the qualitative work they recommend is expensive and time consuming. Nevertheless, we can accept Alexandrova's general point, namely, that the FDA, ISPOR, and others take patients to be experts on their quality of life and because they are so taken, the FDA and others believe that patients' beliefs about these constructs should be sought out and prioritized.

What is wrong with prioritizing patients' perspectives when developing and modifying questionnaires? Part of the problem, Alexandrova (2017, 135) argues, is that by prioritizing patients' perspectives, other considerations regarding the construct might be discounted. Philosophical considerations, for instance, will tend to be discounted as well as considerations from clinicians, psychologists, social workers, and others. In fact, Alexandrova's complaint seems to be that patients are not the relevant experts, and in taking them to be such, we've prioritized the wrong perspectives. This point comes out most clearly when she (2017, 138) discusses a recommendation made by Henrica de Vet (2011), a member of the Vrije Universiteit team who developed the quality criteria I discussed above. In a textbook the VU team published in 2011, they argue that content validity should be determined by experts in the relevant area of medicine. Alexandrova (2017) strongly agrees that a panel of experts is perhaps the best authority on an instrument's content validity. But whereas de Vet and colleagues populate the expert panel with patients from the target population, Alexandrova (2017, 138) populates it with experts in social work, psychotherapy, psychology, economics, sociology, anthropology, and philosophy.[2]

Certainly, Alexandrova (2017, 138) agrees, researchers should check to see if their questionnaires are comprehensible to patients—after all, patients need to be able to understand the questions asked. But when it comes to determining the relevance of a question for measuring, for example, quality of life, patients are not experts. As Alexandrova (2017, 136) puts the point, there are better and worse theories of well-being, and using patient reports to validate these measures denies this fact. Conversational evidentiary subjectivism doesn't take a theory of the construct into consideration when choosing what questions to include; only patients' views serve as evidence. Without a theory to guide the choice of questions, these questionnaires can go badly wrong since, as Alexandrova (2017) points out, we know that people make poor judgments about what is good for them; that is, patients can be wrong about what is part of a good-quality life. This danger is compounded because, she (2017, 143) argues, in questionnaire design there is little effort to mitigate poor judgments or find out what people actually value, as opposed to what they say they value. Using patients' points of view to validate the content of a questionnaire seems to ignore important a priori theoretical constraints or allowances that give shape to a genuinely good quality of life.

Alexandrova's (2017) criticism becomes sharper when we take account of the role she gives theory in her philosophy for a science of well-being. Alexandrova distinguishes mid-level theories from high-level theories. High-level theories are the philosophically familiar, all-things-considered prudential theories of well-being, the "Big Three": hedonism, desire fulfillment, and objective list. Mid-level theories, however, are context-specific, some-things-considered well-being. Some examples might include quality of life in epilepsy or quality of life of people with incontinence. She argues that mid-level theories can better direct the choice of a construct than high-level theories can because they are more specific and more grounded in relevant empirical facts. This means that she thinks mid-level theories are more useful to social scientists. To be more useful, mid-level theories need to move among scientific facts, expert opinion, and abstract philosophical theories.

To illustrate how mid-level theories should work, Alexandrova (2017, 54–76) uses the example of childhood well-being. She begins by taking account of expert beliefs about childhood well-being with an eye toward using these beliefs as constraints on philosophical theories. Experts believe that objective indicators are important for measuring child well-being, and that the concept of development is key to understanding childhood. Alexandrova (2017, 62–68) uses these and other beliefs to test different philosophical theories: ideal subjectivism is set aside largely due to the importance it gives subjective indicators; Richard Kraut's developmentalism, a type of objective list theory, however, is pursued in part because it makes room for what development experts understand as important to childhood well-being.

According to Alexandrova, then, conversational evidentiary subjectivism has two problems: it uses the wrong experts and it avoids considerations of prudential theory. In what follows I will challenge both of these criticisms. Patients, I will argue, are relevant experts for contributing to patient-centered constructs. Patient-centered measures should prioritize patient involvement. Moreover, although I think philosophy has a role to play in validating these measures, this role is not in applying prudential theories of well-being to specific contexts; rather, the role is to articulate an epistemic theory that governs the contributions patients and others make.

3.3. Patients as Epistemic Agents

I think it is fair but unfortunate to say that modern healthcare is known for marginalizing patients. As I have argued previously, patient-centered measures aim to undo some of this marginalization. In this section I explore different ways in which people with disabilities, patients, and other ill persons are epistemically marginalized to clarify the role patient-centered measures have in "capturing patient perspectives" or "representing patient voices."

In her book *Illness as Metaphor* Susan Sontag (1978, 3) famously describes the human condition:

> Everyone who is born holds dual citizenship, in the kingdom of the well and in the kingdom of the sick. Although we all prefer to use only the good passport, sooner or later each of us is obliged, at least for a spell, to identify ourselves as citizens of that other place.

It is nearly impossible, Sontag notes, to enter into the kingdom of the sick without being prejudiced by the "lurid" metaphors describing it. Disease and illness, Sontag argues, are used and understood through metaphors. Cancer is militarized and tuberculosis romanticized. We might note that the metaphors do not stop there: disability is taken to be an obstacle, pregnancy is precarious, conditions such as fibromyalgia and chronic pain are fictionalized, and all of it is medicalized. These metaphors, and the narratives in which we find them, are the dominant cultural resources through which those in the kingdom of the well understand those who are sick or disabled. If you are diagnosed with cancer, you become a fighter, battling the disease; if you are paralyzed, you become brave and long-suffering in the face of undeniable misfortune (Barnes 2016); if you are pregnant, your health is a risk, if you are chronically tired and in pain, your complaints are suspicious.

These narratives are powerful, but their power lies not in furthering our understanding of illness, disease, or disability. In fact, a good deal of their power lies in their ability to obscure our understanding. In Elizabeth Barnes's (2016) excellent monograph *The Minority Body*, she argues that dominant disability narratives function as an identity prejudice. Identity prejudice is a term introduced by Miranda Fricker (2007) to refer to associations between a social group and certain attributes. In the context of illness, disease and disability, identity prejudices function very similarly to Sontag's metaphors. When metaphors such as "disability as misfortune" and the "disabled as plucky overcomers" (Barnes 2016, 142) fill the collective social imagination, they function as identity prejudices: people with disability are unfortunate, yet plucky overcomers.

As Fricker (2007) and Barnes (2016) point out, these metaphors, or identity prejudices as they refer to them, go on to play a role in establishing one's credibility as a knower. When people with disabilities express satisfaction with their lives, when they admit to happiness and describe themselves as having a good life—not happiness and a good life despite their disability, but just happiness and a good life (Barnes 2016, 138)—the tendency is to discount their testimony. If we already know that disability is a misfortune, and if we already know that people with disabilities are brave and stoic in the face of their misfortune, then this "knowledge" explains (away) their testimony. We think: they are so brave; they have overcome so much, they don't even recognize how limited their lives are. When we don't take testimony seriously, we are committing testimonial injustice—we're discounting the

testimony of people with disabilities when we wouldn't discount similar testimony if it was made by people without disability (Barnes 2016).

It isn't simply people with disability who experience testimonial injustice;
it is also a chronic problem in healthcare. The evidence is overwhelming.
Patient narratives (Thomas 2018), empirical evidence (Beckman and Frankel
1984), policy initiatives (Buist 2014), historical accounts, and philosophical analysis (e.g., Kennedy 2013; Kidd and Carel 2017, 2018) all point in the
same direction: patients' credibility as knowers is discounted. Moreover, as
Ian Kidd and Havi Carel (2017) argue, ill persons are particularly vulnerable
to testimonial injustice because they are subject to negative stereotypes, such
as being cognitively impaired, emotionally overwhelmed, or suffering from
health anxiety. These negative stereotypes undermine the testimonial credibility of patients when they try to describe their symptoms or experience.

Testimonial injustice can lead to hermeneutic marginalization. People with
disabilities, patients, and other ill persons are hermeneutically marginalized
when they are excluded from participating in the formation of our collective
understanding. When testimony is discounted as "overly emotional" or "just"
the result of stoicism in the face of misfortune, the understandings that the
testimony articulates are rejected as illegitimate; they aren't taken up as part
of the collective hermeneutical resource about what these experiences can
mean. The result is that part of the significance of losing the ability to walk is
that one's capacity for happiness or one's quality of life decreases, and part of
the significance of being adamant in the face of undiagnosed symptoms or
untreated concerns is that one is too emotional. When hermeneutic marginalization occurs with people with disabilities, patients, and other ill persons,
the concepts, definitions, stories, and so on that we reach for to make sense of
the human world end up being ableist.

When our collective hermeneutic resource is prejudiced in this way, it
affects not only how able-bodied people understand the experiences and
stories of disability and illness, but also self-understanding of those who are
disabled and ill. We can think of this marginalization in terms of the classic
hermeneutic relationship of part and whole that I introduced in Chapter 1;
understanding is a matter of fitting the parts of a text or its analogues, for
instance, human actions, speech, symbols, works of art, into a coherent
whole. Understanding gets started when we project meaning onto the whole
and see how the parts cohere with this meaning. The dominant cultural
understandings of disability and illness as, for example, a medical problem
or a misfortune make it difficult for individuals to make sense of, or even

articulate, their individual experiences that challenge or nuance the dominant understanding.

Hermeneutic marginalization can make the hermeneutic circle of part and whole appear vicious. When happiness or a good-quality life is partly defined in terms of being able to walk, or when rationality is partly defined by deference to authority, it is difficult to articulate an experience that contravenes these definitions. What words could one use to articulate happiness as a quadriplegic that would not be understood as examples of stoicism or denial? What emotions could serve to further the insistence of rational belief and action that would not instead reinforce interpretations of emotional or fraught decision-making? When the experiences of people with disability, patients, and other ill persons are obscured from collective understanding due to a structural identity prejudice affecting the collective hermeneutical resource, then hermeneutic marginalization is also an injustice (Fricker 2007, 155).

Hermeneutic marginalization and injustice are difficult to spot when it isn't your experience being obscured. In fact, this invisibility is a good deal of the problem when the hermeneutic relationship of part and whole appears vicious (Gadamer 2004, 299). What is needed is something to break the cycle of parts being absorbed into the dominant interpretation of the whole; what we need, as I discussed in Chapter 1, is something that will pull us up short by the text, something that will create space for us to recognize our assumptions and values *as* assumptions and values and begin to reason about them. The function of first-person illness narratives and the Disability Pride movement is at least, in part, to do just this.

Since the 1980s AIDS epidemic, first-person illness narratives have proliferated. Arthur Frank (2003) argues that this increase is proof that there is more to the experience of illness than the medical story can provide. To be sure, perhaps there has always been more to the experience of illness than medicine can tell, but post–World War II changes in how medical care is delivered have gone a long way toward hermeneutically marginalizing patients. As medicine has become increasingly institutionalized, patient care and treatment have become increasingly depersonalized and reliant on medical technology. Frank (2003) conceptualizes the changes this move renders to patient care as the shift to the modern experience of illness.

In this modern experience of illness, knowledge of what is happening comes from expert others rather than the patient. Modern medicine consigns patients and their loved ones to waiting rooms and hospital beds while specialists and test results tell them the truth of the matter. The patient's voice is often lost; she is hermeneutically marginalized. But autobiographical illness narratives aim to recover some of what is lost by providing an account from the patient's perspective. Frank (2003) thinks of them as maps, in which patients reject the understanding that the modern illness experience provides and begin to find their own. He also thinks of illness narratives as offering guidance to other ill patients who find themselves voiceless. We might think of illness narratives as attempts to give an alternative interpretation of the whole, one that can effectively contribute to the collective hermeneutic resource.

Barnes (2016, 143–67) argues persuasively that the Disability Pride movement is also a way of acknowledging and disrupting hermeneutic marginalization and injustice. Barnes (2016, 173–78) focuses on prejudices that are based on what she calls normatively laden distinctions. The "misfortunate disabled person" is normatively laden, she argues, while "dumb blond" is descriptive. The distinction, Barnes believes, lies in whether or not we can undermine the prejudices with counterexamples. I give you a list of intelligent blond women and the veracity of your prejudice about blonds being unintelligent seems to fail. But with normatively laden prejudices, Barnes argues, counterexamples seem to work to reinforce the prejudice.

I'm not concerned with whether Barnes's distinction between descriptive and value-laden prejudices can be defended. I am interested, however, in the phenomenon that her value-laden prejudices describe. The outcome of these value-laden prejudices is what I refer to above as the vicious hermeneutic circle. If counterexamples don't work to combat these kinds of prejudices, then, Barnes argues, we need a different strategy. We need to disrupt radically the collective understanding in a way that turns it on its head; or, I suggested above, we need an alternative interpretation of the whole. Disability Pride does this by celebrating the very features that the collective hermeneutic resource understands as tragic, sad, shameful, serious, regretful, and so on. In celebrating these features, Barnes argues, Pride movements are a way of demanding epistemic justice by insisting that our collective hermeneutic resource accommodate understandings that people with disability have of themselves.

Disability Pride is a striking and clever platform for illustrating the deficiencies of our collective hermeneutic resource. When people with disabilities take to the streets en masse, they provide an alternative interpretation of disability in a vehicle that is difficult to dismiss or explain away. Pride parades do not simply offer a part of the puzzle that we must configure into our larger understanding; rather, they project an interpretation of the whole and challenge non-disabled experiences to fit into *it*. Illness narratives achieve something similar, not as individual books, but, again, en masse, as a recognized genre of literature. Pride parades and illness narratives present stark questions to non-disabled, non-ill, non-patient populations: What if disability is a continuum and we are all limited by our bodies? What if health is temporary and fleeting? What if happiness and a good-quality life do not have reliable physical contributions? What if medicine promises more than it can ever deliver? What if the non-disabled, non-ill, and non-patient populations don't know enough about disability and illness to say very much about it?

These questions demand answers. Individual patients on a ward can be ignored and marginalized, individuals with disabilities can be caricaturized and thus ignored and marginalized, but collective action in the form of Pride parades, and the critical mass of published books on first-person experiences with illness, demand acknowledgment. We might say that Pride movements and illness narratives can make this demand because they provoke our assumptions or prejudice. In provoking them, these prejudices are suspended, and the work they do is delayed. Hermeneutic marginalization and injustice, which was difficult to spot, is now at least partially set in relief. A space for recognition and reasoning is created. The structure of this provocation is the question. In *Truth and Method* (Gadamer 2004, 355) writes that the first condition of understanding, as opposed to misunderstanding, is when someone or something addresses us. We recognize that we are beginning to understand when a text or its analogue raises questions for us—as I suggest Pride movements and illness narratives successfully do.

3.4. An Epistemic Theory for Patient-Centered Measures

What does this discussion of epistemic injustice have to do with patient-centered measures? It does two things. First, this discussion clarifies what I take "capturing patient perspectives" and "representing patients' voices" to mean. People with disabilities, patients, and other ill persons—the very populations patient-centered measures are intended to serve—commonly suffer from identity prejudices that affect their ability to be heard, believed, and understood. This phenomenon is widespread and difficult to overcome, but it is not new. Part of the reason we have something called "patient-centered care" is that clinicians and others recognize this problem and seek to overcome it. If patient-centered measures are going to be worthy proxies for patient perspectives, they cannot reinforce identity stereotypes. Similar to Pride movements and illness narratives, patient-centered measures should incorporate constructs that accommodate understandings that people with disabilities, patients, and other ill persons have of themselves.

Second, the discussion of epistemic injustice helps us to see that the issues at stake in patient-centered measures are not only ethical or moral, but also epistemic. Similar to any measuring instrument, their aim is to translate empirical content into theoretical significance. They are supposed to tell us what the answers on questionnaires mean in terms of a knowledge claim about the construct of interest. But recall also from Chapter 1 that patient-centered measures lack coordination—they lack a link between the constructs we want to measure and our empirical measuring procedures, and this is largely because we lack construct theories.

My suggestion, following on from the discussion in Section 3.3, is that people with disabilities, patients, and other ill persons should be our primary partners in coming to understand patient-centered constructs and developing conceptual frameworks. I make this suggestion not simply because I think it enhances trust, but because living in the "kingdom of the sick" puts patients in a position to teach us something; their standpoint gives them expert knowledge (Harding 1986). Happily, this suggestion dovetails with recent emphasis on content validity: patients' perspectives should be prioritized when determining the content of patient-centered constructs. But the largely qualitative criteria the FDA and ISPOR recommend for content validity are not sufficient for what I have in mind, not for the ethical or epistemic dimension of these measures. Patient-centered measures need a theory to govern patient contributions to the development of measurement constructs and conceptual frameworks. The theory that philosophy can provide, and the theory patient-centered measures need, is not a construct theory or a theory of prudential value, but an epistemic theory that governs patient and other contributions to the construct and its conceptual framework.

We need this epistemic theory to forestall two practical concerns. The first concern is articulated in Alexandrova's (2017) criticism of conversational evidentiary subjectivism, namely, that relying on people with disability's, patients', and other ill persons' testimony may lead to an uncritical acceptance of the content of our constructs. If patient-centered measures prioritize patient involvement, what happens if patients endorse or ignore factors that others feel strongly should or should not be included? Must we always acquiesce to patients' points of view? In other words, must patients' views silence others just as they have been silenced? The second concern worries that even if we say we want to rely on patients to understand our constructs, our procedures may be ossified and unable to incorporate new, and perhaps unusual, points of view. This concern speaks to the motivation of my second patient-centered criterion: patient-centered measures must be inclusive. An epistemic theory is needed for patient-centered measures to manage two kinds of concerns, an anything-goes concern and a concern that only the familiar will be heard. I will address the anything-goes concern in the remainder of this chapter, and the ossification concern in the next.

3.4.1. Epistemic and Ethical Harm: Quality of Life with Epilepsy

In this section I begin to develop an epistemic theory for patient-centered measures. My focus will be on my claim that patient-centered measures should prioritize the involvement of people with disabilities, patients, and other ill persons, and the associated worry that in giving them this power we may slide into uncritical acceptance of their points of view. Before beginning, however, it is important to flag two roles that people with disabilities, patients, and other ill persons can play in the research into patient-centered measurement: a developmental role and a respondent role.

People with disabilities, patients, and other ill persons can work with researchers in the development and modification phase of patient-centered measures to create the content of the target constructs. This includes but is not limited to generating items and response options, developing a conceptual framework, and identifying ethical, social, and other values important in the consideration of the construct. This developmental role is similar to the role the FDA and ISPOR give patients in the context of content validity. In this role, people with disabilities, patients, and other ill persons are crucial in determining how the construct is initially understood and operationalized in the measure.

A second role that members of these populations play is as respondents to the questionnaire. In this role people with disabilities, patients, and other ill persons provide measurement indications by answering questions about their functioning, symptoms, affective state, satisfaction, and so on. These indications are used by researchers to underwrite claims about the target construct, for instance, physical functioning, mobility, upper-arm functioning, and quality of life. My focus in this chapter is with the first role people with disability, patients, and other ill persons play, while the second role will be the focus of the next chapter.

In Chapter 2, I discussed Leplège and Hunt's (1997) argument in their article "The Problem of Quality of Life in Medicine." While they applaud efforts to give prominence to the views and experiences of patients, they argue that asking patients to respond to questions designed by medical experts is not sufficient to claim that the outcomes reflect patients' viewpoints. The example they give is questionnaires designed to measure quality of life in patients with epilepsy. Leplège and Hunt (1997, 49) point out that these measures tend to have content that focuses on frequency and severity of seizures, physical functioning, and paid employment. But the qualitative research on people with epilepsy shows that they are primarily concerned with the stigma associated with having epilepsy and the need to conceal their condition: "Severity and frequency of seizures are of much less concern." As Leplège and Hunt (1997, 49) put it, the problem with these measures and others like them is that they do little more than "force patients to address themselves to the concerns of physicians and/or social scientists and statisticians."

What is the harm in asking patients to address the concerns of clinicians and researchers? After all, neurologists have relevant clinical expertise of epilepsy and patients with epilepsy, as well as the kinds of treatments for epilepsy and their side effects. Socials scientists and statisticians have relevant expertise in questionnaire design. Why aren't patient answers to clinical and researcher questions enough to reasonably claim that we've represented patient perspectives? Could we not understand "patient perspectives" to refer to patient perspectives to clinician questions? In the previous section I dealt with this question in a general sense; in what follows I want to address it specifically in the context of patient centered constructs.

First, I address the epistemic question: When patients give answers to questions developed by clinicians and researchers, why isn't this sufficient to justify the representation of patient perspectives? As I discussed in the previous section, by many accounts, hermeneutic marginalization and injustice are widespread within populations of people with disabilities, patient, and other ill persons. Members of these populations are often excluded from participating in the formation of our collective understanding, and this

exclusion is sometimes due to identity prejudices. One consequence of hermeneutic marginalization and injustice is that the experiences of people with
disabilities, patients, and ill persons are misunderstood by others. When
the non-disabled, non-patients, and non-ill persons develop questions for
patient-centered measures, we should expect these misunderstandings to ex-
tend into the questions posed.

Let's look at an example. What collective hermeneutic resources are readily
available for understanding epilepsy? In *Representing Epilepsy* Jenette Stirling
(2010), discusses understandings of epilepsy from the late 19th century to
the present. She begins with a contemporary account, taken from an install-
ment of the BBC's *Brain Story* in which temporal lobe epilepsy is presented as
a physical process of the brain that can impact thought processes, emotions,
and perception. The documentary incorporates three stories of epilepsy, two
told from the perspective of medical researchers and one from the perspective of a patient. Stirling (2010, xiv) writes that in *Brain Story* we encounter a
150-year-old epilepsy narrative, one nearly as long as the study of neurology
itself. In this narrative, epilepsy is understood as a physical state that demands
medical intervention, but also, insofar as it produces enhanced sensory
experiences, one that can be understood as a talent of sorts. Yet in reading
her account, we can see that the talent is perilous, producing intensely pleas-
urable sensory experiences that are understood in a variety of moral hues.
Stirling examines this variety through the representation of characters with
epilepsy in literature and film. She describes epileptic characters as imbued
with violence, criminality, sexual transgression, artistic genius, and spiritual
insight. Even if some of these representations have positive connotations,
like van Gogh's genius, they are, nonetheless, representations of a mysterious,
not wholly rational, not wholly in-control Other.

When people without epilepsy think about how epilepsy affects those
who have it—perhaps by imagining how it would most affect them if they
did have it—they consider it in terms of the meaning it has for them. This
meaning will come from personal experiences with those who have epilepsy
or from collective hermeneutic resources. As Stirling (2010) discusses, the
medical epilepsy narrative largely understands epilepsy as a physical process
that demands medical intervention. Epilepsy is defined medically (Brodie
and French 2000) by seizures, and medical treatment aims to control them.
It is not surprising that clinicians would understand epilepsy's affect in terms
of the severity and frequency of seizures—as they did in the quality of life
questionnaires Leplège and Hunt discuss.

As Stirling (2010, xvii–xxi) also discusses, the medical narrative recognizes the enhanced sensory experiences that sometimes accompany epilepsy. How might these experiences affect one's life? Our collective hermeneutic resource understands these experiences as manifesting in a variety of ways, but it is consistent in expressing caution. These sensory experiences can be unpredictable. In light of this, it is not surprising to find questions of physical functioning and employment included in measures focusing on quality of life with epilepsy. Such questions help non-epileptic people determine, in a neutral way, whether such sensory experiences negatively affect one's life. This approach to quality of life is reminiscent of the capability approach, which I discussed in the previous chapter.

What is epistemically problematic with using patient answers to these kinds of questions to ground a claim about patient perspectives? Questions in patient-centered measures presuppose the relevance of their subject matter. When a patient-centered measure asks about recent employment history or physical functioning, these questions presuppose that frequency of seizures, recent employment history, and physical functions are the central factors, or central proxy factors, that affect the construct, in this case quality of life. Qualitative research on people with epilepsy, however, suggests that while seizures are relevant, stigma, discrimination, prejudice, and lack of support are equally, if not more, important to quality of life.

Consider: in a systematic review of qualitative studies of children's experiences with epilepsy, Chong and colleagues (2016) found that adolescent patients with severe, frequent, or uncontrolled seizures dealt with more disempowerment and were less likely than others to delineate epilepsy from their identity. So the frequency and severity of seizures does tell us something about quality of life. For instance, when the frequency and severity of seizures is high, these questions might serve as a proxy for disempowerment. But the study also found that independent of frequency and severity of seizures, children suffered from perceived discrimination, which led to isolation and depression. Moreover, this study's findings concur with others (Fayed et al. 2015) showing that parental and peer support is the most important factor in health-related quality of life in children. Strong support enables children to accept their disease and avoid the isolation and depression that comes when they feel stigmatized by their condition.

In another qualitative study focusing on 24 young people between 13 and 25 years of age, Wilde and Haslam (1996) found that 71% identified themselves as victims of stigma. Moreover, while employment was a significant concern for the majority (71%), the concerns were less about their ability to hold a job than about the ability to become employed once their condition was disclosed. In discussing how they felt about living with epilepsy, two-thirds said their lives were greatly disrupted by epilepsy, but this disruption was understood differently. Four of the respondents found the physical limitations of epilepsy frustrating; others expressed frustration over the limits imposed on them by others and identified encouragement to succeed as vital, although not always forthcoming. Here we see that although physical functioning is not irrelevant, for most interviewees in this study the social limits of epilepsy are more problematic.

The purpose of patient-centered measures is to "capture patient perspectives." When the non-disabled, non-patients, and non-ill people design the questions for patient-centered measures, it is likely the questions will over-represent the concerns of those designing the measures and fail to represent relevant aspects of the construct as understood by populations of people with disabilities, patients, and other ill persons. This epistemic limitation is due to hermeneutic marginalization and injustice. In the case of epilepsy, the questionnaires Leplège and Hunt (1997) discuss focus on seizures, physical functioning, and employment, but they only tell part of the story. When we listen to people with epilepsy, we find that seizures can cause anxiety, disempowerment, and fear, but social stigma is equally, if not more, problematic. Part of the anxiety about having a seizure is that others will see it, one's privacy will be violated, and stigmatization will ensue. Seizures cannot be a simple proxy for anxiety because support seems to mitigate anxiety. Moreover, beyond some upper limit, the frequency and severity of seizures may not correlate with anxiety. Furthermore, employment is important to quality of life, but not having a job because employers imagine you are a liability is qualitatively different from not having a job because your seizures are too frequent and/or severe. Physical functioning matters to quality of life, but support from parents and peers matters even more.

Qualitative research is important in understanding the factors that affect the quality of life of people with epilepsy from their point of view.[3] Indeed, this research opens another side to epilepsy that is typically obscured from the collective hermeneutic resource—and that resource is epistemically poorer for it. To be sure, we could stipulate that patient-centered measures represent patient perspectives insofar as patients simply answer questions, no matter who poses them. But given the example above, it seems more natural to say that in that case patient-centered measures ignore patient perspectives. Moreover, this stipulation would not get us past the fact that qualitative work on people with disability, patients, and ill persons provides insight into the constructs we are interested in pursuing; it enriches our understanding of them. Ignoring what people with disability, patients, and ill persons have to say limits what we know about our constructs. This is epistemically problematic.

The problem, however, is not only epistemic; it is also ethical. It would be disingenuous—in fact, doubly unjust—to report patient responses to questions about seizures and employment as representative of their perspectives on quality of life. People with epilepsy already experience hermeneutic injustice and have historically done so (Stirling 2010; Vaccarella 2011; Fadiman 1997). This is the first injustice: to be excluded from participating in the formation of our collective understanding, to have one's experiences misunderstood, to have trouble articulating one's self-understanding. But it is an additional injustice when these misunderstandings are passed off as voicing patients' perspectives. This is the injustice that patient-centered measures are in danger of perpetuating when patients are not involved in the development and modification of these instruments.

I began this section asking, what is the harm in asking patients to address the concerns of clinicians and researchers? There are at least three. First, in her discussion of the harm of epistemic injustice, Fricker (2007) follows Edward Craig (1990, p. 36) in distinguishing between informants and sources of knowledge. When a person is treated as a source of knowledge, she is objectified to obtain an epistemic end, and, crucially, in doing so her subjectivity is undermined. Alternatively, an informant is a person with whom we enter into the give-and-take of reasons that constitutes knowledge formation. As we have seen, when people with disabilities, patients, and other ill persons answer questions developed by non-disabled, non-patients, and non-ill persons, they are treated as sources of knowledge, not informants. Second, because patient-centered measures claim to capture patients' perspectives or represent patients' voices, respondents' subjectivity is not simply undermined, but effectively silenced. Third, patient-centered measures weaken public trust. As Maya Goldenberg (2016, 2021) has argued regarding vaccine hesitancy, public health and epidemiological science can only be effective if the public largely accepts and follows the claims they make. The same is true of drug-labeling claims and claims of quality of care and effectiveness. Yet accepting and acting on the claims of medical science requires trust; it requires the lay public to have faith that science is reported responsibly. If health policy-makers, the FDA, industry, and so on claim to represent patient perspectives, but instead effectively silence them, they risk the public's trust.

As representations of patient voices, patient-centered measures need to accommodate the understandings that people with disabilities, patients, and other ill persons have of the constructs used to evaluate them. This is both epistemically and ethically necessary. Researchers should prioritize patient involvement in the development of patient-centered measures. But what does this mean in practice? Partly, it means that the FDA is on the right track in requiring extensive qualitative research as evidence of content validity. People with disabilities, patients, and other ill persons should play a developmental role in determining the items for patient-centered measures and developing conceptual frameworks.

Yet qualitative research methods are not sufficient to safeguard against the ethical and epistemic pitfalls of giving patients this role. As Alexandrova (2017) reminds us, people can make poor judgments about what is good for them; people with disabilities, patients, and other ill people can be wrong about what is part of a good-quality life. Our approach to prioritizing patient involvement should take this fact into account. Qualitative research is used to answer questions about experiences and their meaning from a certain perspective. Observational research, in-depth interviews, and focus groups are the three most common methods for answering such questions. But in developing the content of a construct, we are interested not only in the experiences and meanings of a particular population, but also whether these experiences and meanings contribute toward a *better* understanding of the construct (or, alternatively, obscure our understanding). How do we know if the experiences people with disabilities, patients, and other ill persons bring to qualitative research help us to understand or misunderstand? Answering this question means going beyond empirical methods to the ethical and epistemic dimensions of hermeneutic experience.

3.4.2. When Do Experiences Undermine Understanding?

Thus far I've argued that people with disabilities, patients, and other ill persons suffer from hermeneutic marginalization and injustice. I have also argued that the reason this marginalization is epistemically problematic is that patients have an expertise in what it is like to live with their conditions, an expertise that enriches our knowledge of constructs such as quality of life, health status, functioning, symptoms, and so on. But as Alexandrova (2017) notes, this expertise is not infallible. Like any point of view, the conditions that lead to patients' perspectives can also lead to misunderstanding. Examples may be instructive.

Take the practices of female and male circumcision. Imagine that we do in-depth interviews with individuals who have undergone these procedures. The female interviewees are mostly middle-aged Muslim Egyptian women of a variety of socioeconomic backgrounds, and the male interviewees are middle-aged North Americans from a variety of religious and socioeconomic backgrounds. Imagine further that the majority in both groups report positive experiences.[4] The women report circumcision as being important to a healthy marriage, integral to social inclusion and religious life. The men report health benefits, religious obligations, and social and familial inclusion. How should we understand these responses? Do they improve our understanding of circumcision or do they confuse it? Perhaps North American and European researchers are inclined to think that the women's experiences confuse the practice and the men's experiences clarify it. But if this is the case, why is it the case (see, for instance, Svoboda et al. 2016 or Earp 2017)? How should we distinguish the points of view that further our understanding and those that impede it? And how should we do this when our own prejudices may be part of our impediment?

Here is another example. At the beginning of this chapter, I said that in 2012 the FDA began including patient perspectives in the regulatory review process as part of the Patient-Focused Drug Development Program. These perspectives were sought through public disease-specific meetings. Of particular interest is the October 2014 meeting that sought expert patient views on female sexual disfunction (FSD). These meetings followed two failed applications from Sprout Pharmaceuticals (2009 and 2013) for the approval of Addyi (flibanserin), a drug for pre-menopausal hypoactive sexual desire disorder. The applications failed because the FDA was unconvinced the evidence demonstrated a positive risk/benefit ratio. The third application (2015) was successful. The evidence submitted on the drug's efficacy was unchanged from the first two applications, but in this third application, Sprout provided additional safety data that was enough to convince the multidisciplinary advisory committee convened by the FDA and, later, the FDA itself that the drug should be approved (Gellad et al. 2015). By some lights the new safety data was thin, and some philosophers (Homan and Geislar 2018) have argued that the re-evaluation of the risk/benefit ratio for flibanserin was due more to the outcomes of the public meeting than this new evidence. My interest here is not whether this public meeting had the influence over approval some have suggested, but rather to use this meeting to illustrate why testimony from people with disabilities, patients, and other ill people needs to be supplemented with critical dialogue from other interested parties.

In their article "Sex, Drugs and Corporate Ventriloquism: How to Evaluate Science Policies Intended to Manage Industry-Funded Bias," Bennet Holman and Sally Geislar (2018) analyze the transcripts from the FDA's public meeting about flibanserin. They argue that industry-sponsored participants were able to capture the meeting and alter its outcome. In their analysis Holman and Geislar identified 19 of the 33 participants as individuals affiliated with Sprout Pharmaceuticals. This affiliation was discovered through disclosed paid travel expenses (n = 16), and Holman and Geislar's (2018, 872) independent discovery of financial relationships (n = 3). Using grounded theory, Holman and Geislar (2018, 873) show that all participants to the meeting (industry and non-industry sponsored) shared a common experience of "total lack of sexual desire." Yet, how this experience was understood differed perfectly between the industry-affiliated group and the non-industry-affiliated group. The industry-affiliated group understood the experience as a biological problem needing medical treatment. The non-industry-affiliated group understood it as a relationship problem that could be dealt with through counseling and behavioral therapy. Moreover, while both groups offered a feminist critique of FSD, those without industry funding discussed the problem in terms of unrealistic expectations of female sexuality. The industry-affiliated group expressed their critique in terms of the FDA's sexism. Men with sexual dysfunction can get a prescription for an FDA approved drug—why can't they?

The FDA's 24-page summary of these meetings, Holman and Geislar (2018, 875) note, uses quotations from industry- and non-industry-affiliated women proportional to their speaking time. Even though industry-affiliated women outnumbered (n = 19) and out-spoke (73%) non-industry-affiliated women, the FDA included a balanced summary of the views expressed. Yet in the summary the FDA effectively ignores the fact that most of the women are industry affiliated. The report only notes in passing that "some participants voluntarily disclosed that their travel to the meeting was funded." Holman and Geislar (2018, 876) argue that by effectively ignoring the significance of industry funding, it was easy for the FDA's subsequent condensing of these meetings to interpret them as a single point of view with minor variations. For instance, in the executive summary of the preparatory briefing document for the advisory committee, "The only mention of the Patient Meeting is a report that women conveyed a willingness to risk serious (and often unknown) adverse effects and even to undergo periodic minor surgery with its related risk of serious infection in order to obtain [FSD] relief" (Holman and Geislar 2018, 876–77). In the live presentations to the advisory committee, industry was able to argue truthfully and effectively that patients themselves had spoken of a need for, and in support of approving, flibanserin. As Holman and Geislar (2018, 77) observe, by the time it was said and done, the voices of non-industry-affiliated women had been silenced.

3.4.3. A Dialogic Account

For the sake of argument, I'm going to assume initially that in the cases above something about the experiences of middle-aged Muslim Egyptian women and the industry-affiliated women has corrupted their understanding of female circumcision and flibanserin, respectively. I'm going to assume, again for the sake of argument, that we take the experience of circumcised men and non-industry-affiliated women not to be corrupted and instead believe their testimony provides greater understanding of male circumcision and flibanserin, respectively. Given these temporary assumptions, I want to ask a question: What do we mean when we say that we have a better or greater understanding of something? When we say that men's experiences with circumcision give us a better understanding of it, what does that mean?

To begin, I want to suggest it means we understand better what male circumcision *is*. Equally, when we misunderstand something, or when we say that testimony obscures understanding, what we mean is that the object of our understanding, say female circumcision or flibanserin, is not as clear as it could be. To put this point philosophically, we can say that understanding has positive (or negative) ontological consequences (Gadamer 2004). Furthering this point, when the women with hypoactive sexual desire disorder give testimony about their experiences, I suggest we think of them as providing more or less explicit interpretations of their disorder. These interpretations can be more or less illuminating in coming to understand what flibanserin is. In underlining this point: there is a distinction between the testimony or interpretation about, say, a drug and the drug itself. They are two different phenomena.

Nonetheless, these phenomena are related. Flibanserin does not come into our "context of concerns," as Georgia Warnke (2011, 8) puts it, as an isolated material object awaiting interpretation. Rather, "We are always already immersed in everyday concerned involvements" with the objects of our interpretation—when we encounter flibanserin, we are already immersed in and familiar with pharmaceuticals, with sex, with sexual desire or its lack, with relationships, with industry, with what it means to take women seriously, and with a historical tradition handed down from one generation to the next (Warnke 2011, 9). Put otherwise, we come to flibanserin and circumcision with a practical pre-understanding of them. This is where we must begin in our understanding of what they are.

Unfortunately, sometimes our pre-understandings seem to overwhelm our subject matter. Earlier I argued that hermeneutic injustice can manifest when the hermeneutic circle turns vicious. For instance, when happiness or a good-quality life is partly understood in terms of being able to walk, or when rationality is partly understood by deference to authority, it is difficult to articulate an experience that contravenes these understandings. What words could one use to articulate happiness as a quadriplegic that would not be understood as an example of stoicism or denial? I argued, however, that illness narratives and Pride movements were ways to break this vicious understanding of parts in terms of the whole. I have further argued that patient-centered measures must also find a way of interrupting the interpretation of parts in terms of the whole—patient-centered measures should not perpetuate identity stereotypes.

Part of the solution to avoid identity stereotyping in patient-centered measures, I have suggested, is to give people with disabilities, patients, and other ill persons a developmental role. But this solution is not as simple as it first seemed. In this developmental role, patients participate in qualitative research. On the one hand, qualitative research is useful because it allows us to foreground minority experiences and their meaning from the whole. This methodology is important because, similar to Pride movements and illness narratives, it offers an opportunity to suspend our everyday assumptions or prejudices and allow the research to raise questions about our own pre-understandings. Simply put, qualitative research allows us to hear patients' voices.

Yet, on the other hand, listening to the testimony of people with disabilities, patients, and other ill persons, although necessary, is not sufficient to secure our epistemic or ethical responsibilities. Testimony is invaluable, but it is not infallible. Some experiences, whether they happen to people with or without disabilities, patients or not, can corrupt our understanding rather than further it. Thus, even when we foreground the testimony of people with disabilities, patients, and other ill persons—as is the aim of qualitative research—we must still evaluate it as improving upon our understanding or obscuring it. And importantly, we cannot escape this evaluative role. Does the experience of circumcised men and women help us to understand or misunderstand circumcision? What kinds of experiences should give us pause in the FDA public meetings? Health researchers will ultimately have to decide how to understand and operationalize patient-centered constructs. Even if people with disabilities, patients, and other ill persons could take over measure development, they would still have to evaluate testimony and interpretations from one another, from old measures, and from clinicians and health researchers, to determine those that help understand the construct and those that cause us to misunderstand.

How should this evaluation proceed? In *Truth and Method*, Gadamer (2004) is well aware of the difficulty: we must evaluate the interpretations of others while recognizing that our own understanding of the topic at hand is far from secure. What should we do? In his discussion of hermeneutic experience Gadamer considers three modes of understanding. In the first mode, we approach another person in the same way we approach an event; that is, we try to understand others to predict their behavior. Within this relationship the person one is trying to understand is objectified, and the point of understanding is to uncover empirical regularities. This is the mode of understanding most often used in medicine: patients are reduced to their bodies, and clinicians probe those bodies, hoping to understand empirical regularities to make a diagnosis and a determine a prognosis (McClimans 2016). Gadamer refers to this as understanding of human nature. As I hope I've made clear, this is not the appropriate mode of understanding for patient-centered constructs.

In the second mode of understanding we consider the subjectivity of others. In considering their subjectivity we listen as others tell their story, we take them at their word, and we try to empathize. We try to understand as they do. But by imagining that by listening to another, we can understand them as they understand themselves, Gadamer thinks we come to dominate them. We manage this deceit by reflecting ourselves out of the relationship. To understand another as they understand themselves, we must conceive of ourselves as being free from our own past, free from our own prejudices, free from tradition. We are thus deluded into believing that we can understand another in an unprejudiced and unbiased manner. But this is an illusion and a dangerous one at that. Those who do not acknowledge the prejudices at work in their own understanding are still dominated by them. By not recognizing these prejudices, they are perpetuated, and, moreover, we mislead others by calling the understanding that results unbiased. For those who think that listening to patients is a simple solution, the lesson here is that we cannot reflect our way out of the tradition in which we find ourselves. The FDA's emphasis on content validity and qualitative research is not a sufficient mode of understanding for patient-centered measures. Gadamer's (2004) criticism of this second mode of understanding is a variation on the concern that Alexandrova has for conversational evidentiary subjectivism. Both are concerned that unexamined assumptions and values will mask themselves as knowledge. Alexandrova is worried that respondents can be wrong about what is important; Gadamer is worried that researchers will espouse concerns in the name of, say, patients, only to further their own assumptions and values.

In Gadamer's third and favored mode of understanding, the aim is to acknowledge the role assumptions and values have in making knowledge possible, while at the same time being ready for these assumptions and values to reveal themselves so we might examine their validity. How do we become ready for this revelation? We do so by preparing for the "otherness" of another person. This means that we should be prepared for another person to "really say something to us" (Gadamer 2004, 361); we should try to understand how what another person says about a subject matter—be it circumcision, flibanserin, epilepsy, or upper-arm functioning—could be true. Here again we see the use to which Gadamer puts the epistemic virtue of possible truth, or, as I referred to it in Chapter 1, epistemic humility. Notice we are not trying to understand the conditions that may have led other people to believe what they are saying is true. Gadamer is not interested in history or psychology; he is not interested in the etiology of belief formation or opinion, but rather epistemology—what *is* the benefit of flibanserin? What *are* the benefits, if any, of male and female circumcision? In taking seriously the truth of another person's testimony, Gadamer believes, our assumptions and values will be provoked and questions will naturally arise as we try to adjust our own understanding to make sense of these new interpretations. As I said earlier, the structure of provocation is the question. Thus, we might ask about the role female circumcision plays in social inclusion. Or how can it promote healthy marriages when it often seems to adversely affect women's sexual health? We might also ask what role the discussion of female circumcision plays in furthering Western dominance. These questions expose our own biases—prioritizing equality and sexual health—while also seeking genuine clarification on what social inclusion and a healthy marriage might mean, as well as what role the West should play in this conversation.

It is through asking questions, receiving answers, and in turn responding to questions posed by others that we work toward a better understanding of the subject matter. Gadamer conceives of this third mode of understanding as dialogical. Warnke (2011, 13) puts it best when she writes:

> Our openness to the otherness of what others say reflects an interest in the possible legitimacy of their claims and our interest in the possible legitimacy of their claims requires the sorts of conversations in which we explore possibilities, compare values and arguments, consider alternative world views and so on. Dialogue or conversation for Gadamer is not, therefore, a process of arguing or trying to find only the errors in the opinions and views of others in an effort to reassert the validity of our own.

The point of what I call *epistemic dialogue* is thus not to argue with others or to become self-satisfied with our own position, but rather to offer provocation in the form of questions so we can foreground and examine our own assumptions and values. But if the point of epistemic dialogue is to provide opportunities for critical reflection, then, as Warnke (2011) recognizes, not just any interlocutors will do. Conversing with those whose assumptions and values are like our own will usually fail to offer provocation. Epistemic dialogue requires that we seek out those who are different from us because they are the ones whose positions are best placed to put our own assumptions and values into question.

Some interpretations help us to understand better, some cause us to misunderstand; for Gadamer determining which is which requires dialogue oriented toward agreement about the subject at hand. Why agreement? For Gadamer an orientation toward consensus provides the appropriate motivation for interlocutors to take each other seriously. If agreement is the goal, I can't simply dismiss positions different from my own and move on; I must instead answer them. But as Warnke discusses, if difference and disagreement are the conditions for critical reflection—for pulling us up sort—doesn't agreement eliminate these conditions? Yes and no. For Gadamer, agreement about the subject matter is more of an aspiration than a goal. It shapes our orientation toward epistemic dialogue in that it gives us reason to take others seriously. But Gadamer doesn't think of agreement as a permanent condition. In fact, he writes, "It is enough to say that we understand in a *different* way, *if we understand at all*" (2004, 297). There are for Gadamer infinite ways in which we will disagree, particularly as we move through time. Nonetheless, Warnke is concerned about those who suffer from dogmatism and extremism right now; in the present. A hermeneutics that relies on the historical timeline to supply the differences for critical reflection is cold comfort to those who are marginalized and harmed here and now. Thus, instead of hermeneutics oriented toward agreement, she argues for a hermeneutics oriented toward impact. This orientation is geared toward understanding how what others understand or say impacts our own views. Impact, Warnke argues, can provoke questions, and thus illuminate our assumptions and values without the need for agreement.

Whether oriented toward agreement or impact, dialogic understanding is not a methodology to follow; it is, rather, a practice to hone. What matters is that I take others seriously as making claims about the possible truth of a subject matter; I practice epistemic humility. I ask questions to understand better, and in turn I am asked questions. We try to work out the impact of our different points of view (or perhaps we come to an agreement, albeit for Gadamer, a contingent one). Sometimes in this process I come to see how I was shortsighted. I see that joy and humor are compatible with disability. My understanding is transformed by thinking of us all as limited by our bodies. Other times I am pulled up short. I have trouble understanding the difference between male and female circumcision in contexts such as in the United States. Or perhaps as a member of the FDA's public meetings on FSD I become convinced that hypoactive sexual desire disorder is partly a biological disorder. These understandings to which I contribute may turn out to be mistaken. For over 200 years European Americans understood African Americans as less than human. They were wrong. Although fallible, epistemic dialogue may be the best we have for securing our epistemic and ethical obligations.

This idea is not a minority point of view. Ethically, the give-and-take of reasons that constitutes knowledge production is also characteristic of epistemic dialogue. In addition, epistemic dialogue characterizes the role of the informant. Recall from earlier that Fricker (2007) favorably contrasts informants with "sources of knowledge." When individuals are treated as sources of knowledge, they are objectified and used as a means to some epistemic end. Informants, however, are treated as subjects with equal standing, and as such their testimony is taken seriously. Taking testimony seriously does not mean accepting it without examination; rather it means considering it, trying to make sense of it and asking questions. This is also what epistemic dialogue requires.

Moreover, we see an epistemic point about dialogue made in Anke Bueter and Saana Jukola's (2020) discussion of the FDA's public meetings on FSD. They too discuss the influence of the industry-affiliated women at the October 2014 meetings. Like Holman and Geislar (2018), they lament the lack of transparency over the financial ties of the participants. But in addition, they suggest that the participants in these meetings should be encouraged to respond to arguments made by other discussants. They argue that "providing such an institutional framework and incentives for critical discourse has the potential to work as a safeguard against bias" (Bueter and Jukola 2020, 467). Furthermore, as Dalal et al. (2010) found in their cross-sectional study of 9,159 Egyptian women, those who attended discussions of female circumcision at community meetings, churches, or mosques, as well as those exposed to knowledge of the health risks, were more likely to support its discontinuation. This finding raises the possibility that through a dialogue about female circumcision Egyptian women may find the validity of their assumption in favor of it lacking and adjust their understanding of the practice accordingly.

3.5. Conclusion

The FDA's 2009 "Guidance for Industry" was a landmark event in the history of patient-centered measurement. Not only did it signal acceptance by the FDA, but it also signaled an important methodological shift emphasizing content over construct validity. This shift dovetailed with the FDA's understanding of PROMs as "capturing the patient's experience." This shift has significant philosophical implications. If we take seriously the claim that these instruments aim to capture patients' experiences and represent patient voices—and why shouldn't we?—then, philosophically, we are in need of an epistemic theory to govern patient contributions, not a prudential theory of what a good life entails. In this chapter I begin to articulate and defend an epistemic theory for patient-centered measures.

Patient-centered measures should prioritize patient involvement and input. People with disabilities, patients, and other ill persons commonly suffer from testimonial and hermeneutic injustice derived from identity stereotypes. If patient-centered measures are going to be trustworthy proxies of "patient perspectives," they cannot perpetuate identity stereotypes. To this end, people with disabilities, patients, and other ill persons should play a developmental role in determining the content of patient-centered constructs as well as developing conceptual frameworks. The FDA's methodological guidance emphasizing content validity and qualitative research with patient populations is an important and necessary step to ensure that their experience is taken seriously, but it is not sufficient. Qualitative research, at most, describes a process that allows us to foreground patients' experiences and their meaning. But we also need to evaluate testimony as aiding or undermining understanding. I have argued that qualitative research should be supplemented with the practice of epistemic dialogue. Epistemic dialogue allows first- and secondhand perspectives to bear on patient-centered constructs. Importantly, this practice acknowledges that people with disabilities, patients, and other ill persons have expertise we need, but like all humans, they are fallible. Moreover, if Warnke is correct that in hermeneutic dialogue we should seek out those who are most different from us, then bringing first- and secondhand perspectives together to understand constructs such as quality of life and functioning is perhaps our best bet in arriving at content valid measures.

4

Ongoing Coordination

In Chapter 3 I started to develop an epistemic theory for patient-centered measurement. This theory captures two insights I've argued for thus far. First, in Chapter 1 I argued that coordinating our measuring instruments with the constructs we aim to measure means accepting that we don't have assumption or value-free evidence of them. Our best measurement methods and models cannot overcome this fundamental epistemic fact. The path forward is to become comfortable with a certain level of epistemic uncertainty. We must affirm what we know about a construct—and build our measures— while at the same time recognizing that some of what we think we know is probably mistaken and will be replaced as we come to understand better.

The second insight concerns the kind of evidence we should use to inform our understanding of the constructs we want to measure. In Chapter 3 I argued that patient-centered measures should prioritize patient involvement through epistemic dialogue. This means that patient involvement through testimony, qualitative research, and other patient-focused study designs should form the backbone of our evidence base. Patient contributions are not one and done. This follows from the fact that our evidence is never free of assumptions and values. Whatever knowledge patients and researchers bring to construct development, it is at best only partial and incomplete. Indeed, Hagquist (2019) seems to anticipate this point. They stipulate that whenever patient-centered instruments are used in relevantly different contexts than they were initially developed, or if there are other reasons to think patient perspectives have changed, patients will need to be consulted and measuring instruments tweaked.

Yet involving patients in construct development does not mean that we simply acquiesce to whatever they say. The practical application of testimony, qualitative research, and other patient-focused study designs need to incorporate this point. Patient involvement is a negotiation with researchers about what is important about what we want to measure, for instance, what kind of questions we should ask and what response options we should offer. We should assume, full stop, that patients can teach us about these constructs,

Patient-Centered Measurement. Leah M. McClimans, Oxford University Press. © Oxford University Press 2024.
DOI: 10.1093/oso/9780197572078.003.0005

but when something doesn't make sense or seems impractical, researchers should feel free to ask questions. Indeed, this is their responsibility. The point of this negotiation is to come to a better understanding of what is to be measured, not adopt the points of view of others. This negotiation is epistemic dialogue, and will no doubt require the cultivation of shared norms, for instance, accepting uncertainty, recognizing patient testimony as a form of pedagogy, and perceiving questions as a mark of respect rather than critique.

In this chapter I continue to fill out this epistemic theory by asking how patient-centered measures can include a range of respondent answers. How can we ensure that measurement outcomes reflect the varied perspectives that people have, for example, on their physical functioning and quality of life? How can we be sure that our measures are sufficiently nimble to incorporate new, and perhaps unusual, points of view? While in Chapter 3 my discussion focused on the developmental role that people with disabilities, patients, and other ill persons play in creating these measures, in this chapter I focus on the role they play as respondents. This distinction is important and helps to pinpoint the inclusivity I aim to address. In the previous chapter I was concerned with patient-centeredness at the front end of measurement, that is, as we develop instruments. I focused on the role people with disabilities, patients, and other ill persons can play in, for instance, construct development, the selection of items and response options, and the identification of values. In this chapter, however, I'm interested in patient centeredness from the back end of measurement, that is, how we can be inclusive of respondent answers even after items and response options have been selected. As we'll see, respondents can mean different things even when presented with the same questions and answers. Accounting for these differences denotes one important dimension of inclusivity, which I address in this chapter.[1]

Questions are the primary unit of investigation in patient-centered measures. As I argued in Chapter 3, question development is an important part of patient-centered measurement. We can reinforce identity stereotypes, undermine trust, and generally foster instances of injustice if we do not involve people with disabilities, patients, and other ill persons in developing these questions. Yet simply asking the right questions is not enough to justify claims about "capturing patient perspectives" and "representing patient voices." Questions require interpretation. If I ask, "How are you feeling?" you may understand it in any number of ways. You might understand it in terms of your emotional health or your physical health or perhaps in terms of your prospects for winning a match. You might understand the question in terms of your emotional health compared to what it was last year, or compared to other cancer patients, or to what you wish it could be. In fact, over time you may change how you understand this question. You may start off understanding it in terms of your emotional health compared to what it was last year but come to understand it in terms of what it's like compared to other cancer patients.

Respondents' interpretations of questions can lead to problems for patient-centered measures because they affect respondent answers. Consider this question from the SF-36: "In general would you say your health is: (please circle one) excellent, very good, good, fair, poor" (Ware and Sherbourne 1992). Respondents might understand this question in terms of "your health *compared to why you would like it to be*" or *compared to that of others with cancer* or *to others of your own age*. The same person may answer that her health is poor compared to where she'd like it to be, excellent compared to others with cancer, but only fair compared to others her age. When these kinds of differences are generalized over the population responding to the questionnaire, they cause problems for interpreting the clinical significance of outcomes. For cross-sectional studies, these problems arise when comparing a population at a single point in time (Mallinson 2002). In longitudinal studies, respondents may understand the same questions differently over time, and this causes problems for assessing change (Sprangers and Schwartz 1999). How should we conceptualize and handle differences of interpretation in the context of these measures?

Traditionally, these kinds of differences in interpretation have been treated as a source of error (Swartz and Rapkin 2004). But in 1999 Mirjam Sprangers and Carolyn Schwartz began conceptualizing some of these differences, specifically certain differences that occur over time, as a source of knowledge. In doing so they translated the concept of "response shift" from the fields of education and organizational change into the field of quality of life research (Vanier et al. 2018). I discussed response shift a bit in Chapter 2. Response shift is defined as a change in the self-evaluation of a target construct over time (Sprangers and Schwartz 1999). It has been used to explain supposedly counterintuitive findings, such as when respondents' health deteriorates but their self-reported quality of life remains the same. According to response shift theory, this might happen when, for instance, a patient reinterprets what a poor quality of life means. They might start off thinking a poor quality of life is not being able to garden, but as their health deteriorates, they may come to think of it as not enjoying a family meal. Thus, as patients' health deteriorates and they can no longer go outside, they may still report a good quality of life because they can eat dinner with their family. Sprangers and Schwartz (1999) believed that including response shift (rather than treating it as a source of error) would provide a better scientific understanding of how quality of life is affected (or not) by changes in health while also aiding in the development of reliable and valid measures of change. For instance, response shift effects may obscure the results from clinical trials when quality of life outcomes remain the same over time due to respondents' change in their self-evaluation of quality of life. Understanding and, eventually, measuring response shift could help explain when quality of life outcomes do and do not provide evidence of effectiveness as well as improve the psychometric properties of patient-centered measures.

There are far-reaching theoretical and methodological implications for considering at least some differences in interpretation as a source of knowledge. In this chapter I lay out what I take to be the main theoretical ones. For although there is now a rich literature on response shift, the attention to the theoretical implications has been insufficient.[2] To address them adequately we need to shift perspectives; we need to move beyond the norms of the health sciences and psychological measurement, which tend to limit how we frame this phenomenon. In this chapter I do this by focusing on the logic of the questions used in most patient-centered measures. Although questions, or items as they are referred to in the psychometric literature, are centrally important to patient-centered measures, they are given surprisingly little attention compared to issues of population selection, data analysis, and study design (Olsen and IEA European Questionnaire Group 1998; Hagquist 2019). This omission suggests a possible epistemology of ignorance. The epistemology of ignorance suggests that historical and practical approaches to knowledge production can generate ignorance as one of their effects. For instance, Charles Mills (1997) and others (Sullivan and Tuana 2007) have argued that the history of racist oppression has led white people to misinterpret social and political reality. Some examples of this ignorance are that modernity began in Europe and spread outward, that global poverty is separate from Western wealth, and that Black men who are injured or killed by police must do something to elicit police reaction (Alcoff 2007). Similarly, we might think of the history of behaviorism in psychology, and in turn the emphasis on methodology in psychometrics and the health sciences, as producing certain erasures that are in turn productive in furthering these sciences' respective goals, namely using the environment to understand human behavior or quantifying latent variables. To this end, I suggest that the comparative neglect of questions illustrates an erasure in psychometrics to which philosophical attention can shed light.

With the obvious exception of individualized measures, which I discussed in Chapter 2, patient-centered instruments use standardized questions. Thus, a theme that runs through this chapter is standardized questions—why we use them, the assumptions we make when we use them, and whether these assumptions are justified. My argument will be that certain practices of standardization can undermine the alignment between validity and fairness in patient-centered measures, or what I will call "fit for purpose."[3]

4.1. Standardized Questions

4.1.1. Operationalizing Invariance

In this literature, one value nearly synonymous with measurement is invariance. Measurement invariance means that the construct being assessed has the same meaning (or structure) across different groups or on different measurement occasions in the same group (Putnick and Bornstein 2016). For instance, if a measure is invariant across men and women, then the construct has the same meaning for both men and women. If a measure is invariant across time, then it has the same meaning for, say, cancer patients over a six-month period. Measurement invariance is important because it allows for comparisons. If a measure is invariant, then we're comparing apples with apples. If a measure is noninvariant, then meaningful comparisons cannot be made across the groups or time for which it is noninvariant. Noninvariant measures are like comparing apples with oranges.

Most patient-centered measures use standardized questions. So do most math and reading tests. Standardized questions present the same wording and question format to respondents at each time-point to aid in the comparison of scores. The use of standardized questions makes sense against an assumption of invariance. If, all things being equal, a construct has the same meaning across populations and time, then standardizing the questions on a test or questionnaire is a way of operationalizing this expectation. Seen thus, standardization is a choice of method to match the structure of a construct. Against the assumption of invariance, questions that are understood differently than expected are misunderstood and the associated answers are wrong.

Consider, for instance, an example of a standardized question from the Education Development Center. A student is given a rectangle measuring approximately, but not exactly, 1.5 by 2.5 inches. The question asks students, "What is the perimeter of this rectangle? Measure with an inch ruler. Round to the nearest inch" (Goldenberg 2020). The correct answer is 8, but in this case the student answered 10. The student answered 10 because she applied the rounding to each of the measured sides instead of the final answer only. In other words, she understood the part of the question "round to the nearest inch" with *respect to each measurement* instead of with *respect to the final answer*. Her answer is wrong because she misunderstood the question. Our response to this misunderstanding is to correct the student: I see where you went wrong. In math when people say "round," the convention is to round the final result only.

Or consider a standardized question from the Nottingham Health Profile (NHP), a generic patient-centered measure. This measure asks a series of standardized questions, which are presented to respondents as statements with yes or no answers. One question prompts with "I find it hard to reach for things, yes/no." In a study by Donovan et al. (1993) respondents completed the NHP and then discussed the questions and their answers with researchers. One respondent answered yes, she found it hard to reach for things. When she explained her answer she said, "I do find it hard to reach for things, yes, because I am short." Like the example above, this answer is wrong because the respondent misunderstood the question. Our response to this misunderstanding might be something like, "The NHP is interested in whether you find it hard to reach for things with *respect to your health*, not with *respect to your height*."

Contrast these two examples of standardized questions with the following example of an unstandardized question, that is, one that does not presuppose invariance. A couple of years ago I bought my first horse. Recently, he started misbehaving in group jumping lessons. Sometimes he won't listen when I ask him to slow down; sometimes he stops in front of jumps. Considering these problems, I asked more experienced riders, "What should I do when Toni won't listen in lessons?" When I asked this question, what I meant was: What should I *opposed to someone else* do with *respect to my leg, hand, and voice aids* when Toni won't listen in the arena? But most of the answers I got were things like, "Put him on the walker," "Lunge him before you ride," "Make sure you vary his work from day to day," and "Ask someone else to jump him for a couple weeks." These answers surprised me. I was expecting answers like relax your hands and use more leg, turn him in a circle, or give him a flake of the stick.

At first, I didn't understand the answers I got as answers to my question. Lunging him and having someone else ride him didn't tell me what to do when *I* was on top of him in the arena. So I kept asking my question. Then I overheard someone say, "I told her what to do with Toni and she ignored me." What? It brought me up short. I started to reconsider. I had thought my problem with Toni began when I got up on him; I also thought that somehow my riding was the solution to the problem. But if the answers I got were at least partial answers to my question (she ignored me!), then they were telling me that perhaps this was not the best way to understand my question. Instead, these answers seemed to suggest that the problem began before I got up on Toni.

Taking these answers seriously meant reinterpreting my question as something like "What should I *as opposed to someone else* do *with respect to prevention* when Toni won't listen in lessons?" This reinterpretation was helpful. It allowed me to understand the topic of my question more holistically. Riding Toni—or any horse—positively doesn't begin when you get into the saddle for a lesson. These answers helped to remind me of this fact. It also reminded me that when things go wrong, improving my mediocre riding skills is not the only thing I can do. At the same time, this new way of understanding my question didn't wholly respond to my original concern of what I could do *in the saddle*. This concern was still important to me even after considering (and acting on) the alternatives. The upshot is that I didn't simply acquiesce to others' understanding of my question. Instead, I used the answers I received to sharpen the gap in my own understanding and to learn more about my topic. Consequently, the gap in my understanding became more specific: What should I do *in and out of the saddle as opposed to one or the other with respect to prevention* when Toni won't listen in lessons?

Unlike the math and NHP questions, the question about riding Toni wasn't misunderstood in any of its interpretations, nor were any of the proposed answers wrong. Those familiar with van Fraassen's (1980) pragmatic explanation will be appreciate how the different relevance relations and contrast classes created different interpretations of the question with different appropriate answers (McClimans 2011). These different interpretations were sensitive to my interests and the interests of others with more riding experience than me. But neither my interests nor their experience settled the meaning of the question; rather the meaning was negotiated over time as I came to understand my own concerns better through this "dialogue" with others. Moreover, how I understand this question about riding Toni could change in the future if I ask it again (as Toni's behavior, my riding, and my interlocutors change); and it may be understood differently if another person asked it about another horse. In contrast, the math and NHP questions were misunderstood, and the answers given were wrong because when we standardize questions, we implicitly standardize the meaning of the questions.

4.1.2. Standardization: Aiming for Objectivity and Fairness

Standardization is not only a method to operationalize invariance. Often standardization is also aspirational insofar as it seeks to ensure the epistemic and social virtues of objectivity and fairness. By posing the same questions and response options to respondents, standardized questions aid in the objective assessment of the construct under investigation. In the psychometric context, "objective" means respondent answers are caused by the construct, that is, they aren't caused by what are considered irrelevant circumstances or personal idiosyncrasies. For instance, gender, race, ambiguity, social desirability, motivation, and emotional maturity are examples of irrelevance.[4] Psychometric objectivity might fruitfully be understood as mechanical objectivity (Daston and Galison 2007; Reiss 2020). According to Daston and Galison (2010, 120), mechanical objectivity aims to repress interpretation and replace it with procedures that "move nature to the page." Standardized questions aid mechanical objectivity in reducing the interpretations respondents give to questions and the interpretations researchers give to their answers. The hope is that with the correct content, standardized questions will reflect the construct and only the construct, thereby moving "nature to the page" via respondent answers.[5] Mechanical objectivity is related to validity. In fact, it is the handmaid to validity, aiding validity in its quest to measure that which the instrument aims to measure (and nothing else).

Clearly, as I discussed in Chapter 1, validity is important to measurement. Yet as I discussed in Chapter 3, validity is not only an epistemic concern, but also has an ethical dimension. In Chapter 3 I was concerned with the possibility of disingenuous outcomes. Here I want to draw attention to fairness. When measurement outcomes influence resources, diagnoses, ability tracking, and so on—as patient-centered outcomes often do—we are not only interested in validity, but also fairness. Or perhaps a better way to put this is to say that when measurement outcomes are put to these kinds of purposes, then validity is not only of epistemic but also ethical concern. Fitness for purpose requires it. This point is widely recognized. Indeed, *Standards for Education and Psychological Testing* (American Educational Research Association 2014, 49) says, "Fairness is a fundamental validity issue" and devotes an entire chapter to "Fairness in Testing." In what follows I discuss two of the concerns about fairness the *Standards* raises: construct irrelevance and opportunity to learn.

4.2. Construct Irrelevance

Standardized questions support mechanical objectivity. Yet even when questions are standardized, respondents are not standardized. Respondents come to standardized questions as individuals. Their differences—in experience, education, ethnicity, class, gender, and so on, can affect how they answer standardized questions. Irrelevant individual- or group-level differences can undermine objectivity, and when test scores are affected by processes that are extraneous to the test's intended purpose, we call it construct irrelevance (American Educational Research Association 2014, 12). Construct irrelevance is a form of systematic error that can increase or decrease scores of a specific person or a group. It encompasses a broad range of phenomena. Stereotype threat, group membership, irrelevant abilities, and social desirability are among those that can cause construct irrelevance. For instance, individuals may perform differently on a test depending on their preconceived notions of how they will perform (rather than relative to their ability). Or consider a math test with reading problems. If the reading level required to comprehend the math problems gets in the way of doing the math, then this is construct irrelevance. Take a third example. A respondent answering questions for an anxiety measure underreports anxiety because he hopes to appear less anxious (American Educational Research Association 2014, 12–13). This is also construct irrelevance.

No measure is without error. In the face of error researchers seek to minimize and model it. Minimizing construct irrelevance can be achieved by, for instance, taking care to standardize the testing environment or developing well-crafted questions. Yet even the most carefully developed questions and thoughtfully curated testing environments can yield construct irrelevance, so researchers would also like to manage construct irrelevance by modeling it. But it can be difficult to identify construct irrelevance in patient-centered measures. This difficulty stems from the fact that we cannot identify construct irrelevance based on respondent answers or even patterns in their answers. Below I discuss two of these difficulties, a practical difficulty and a theoretical one.

4.2.1. Identifying Construct Irrelevance:
A Practical Problem

Sometimes in measurement we can identify construct irrelevance by looking at incorrect answers. The incorrect answer provides the clue for how the measure's purpose was thwarted by construct irrelevance. For example, recall the math question from earlier: "What is the perimeter of this rectangle? Measure with an inch ruler. Round to the nearest inch" (Goldenberg 2020). The student in this example answered 10. The correct answer is 8. In this case, the student's incorrect answer helps us understand what she did wrong: she rounded each side of the rectangle instead of the final answer only. She didn't understand the convention for rounding. Imagine the primary purpose of this test was to assess knowledge of perimeters rather than knowledge of rounding. A teacher who realizes the source of error may give partial credit for this incorrect answer. Her reasoning is that knowledge of rounding is at least partially irrelevant to the point of the test. Giving partial credit adjusts for construct irrelevance from a validity perspective; it also addresses fairness from a fit for purpose perspective.

Similarly, in the example from the qualitative study of the NHP researchers were able to identify construct irrelevance by working backward from the respondent's answer. Recall the prompt: "I find it hard to reach for things, yes/no." The respondent answered, I do find it hard to reach for things, yes, because I am short. Here the respondent understood the question with *respect to height*, but the intended meaning is *respect to health*. How researchers respond to this respondent's interpretation will depend on the purpose of the qualitative study. In this particular case, Donovan et al. (1993) sought to reveal some of the limitations of generic health status measures. The authors were particularly concerned with how misunderstandings such as this one can cause overestimations of morbidity. Moreover, they were worried about how these kinds of misunderstandings can affect the bigger picture of health-care needs to which these measures contribute. As the authors discuss, the question of healthcare needs is typically linked to policy concerns of ine-quality. Measures that misrepresent morbidity cannot accurately estimate healthcare needs, and thus cannot be used to redress inequality. Thus, in this case, the researchers did not correct the respondent's interpretation of the question. Instead, this interpretation was precisely what the researchers sought in conducting the study.

Qualitative studies such as Donovan et al.'s (see also Mallinson 2002; Westerman et al. 2008) are relatively rare. In the everyday use of patient-centered measures we don't see behind the answers respondents provide. Moreover, unlike most math tests, patient-centered measures don't discrimi-nate among answers. In other words, when respondents are asked if they find it hard to reach for things: yes or no, either answer can be correct (depending on whether they do in fact find it hard to reach for things). Thus, we can't identify incorrect respondent answers *tout court*. Unless looking for them explicitly (Sajobi et al. 2018), we usually discover anomalous respondent answers only when an instrument doesn't correlate well with another instru-ment (CTT) or when there is lack of model fit (Rasch). But as I discuss below, while lack of correlation or model fit may alert us to the possibility of con-struct irrelevance, this claim is often underdetermined by the evidence.

4.2.2. Identifying Construct Irrelevance: A Theoretical Problem

Within psychometrics, construct irrelevance is often associated with differ-ential item functioning (DIF) (Thompson 2018). DIF is a statistical prop-erty of a question. It occurs when different groups or individuals with the same ability level have different probabilities associated with answering a question. For instance, older people may respond differently than younger people to questions about fatigue even after controlling for overall levels of fatigue. But—and this is important—DIF can be benign *or* adverse. If dif-ferent groups or individuals have different probabilities for an item because the question refers to a dimension of the construct that is different for that group or individual, then DIF is benign (Douglas et al. 1996; Breslau et al. 2008). If, however, the different probabilities are because the question taps into something irrelevant to the construct, then it is adverse (Douglas et al.

1996; Breslau 2008 et al.). The mere finding of DIF cannot point us in one direction or the other; it is underdetermined by the evidence.

Determining when DIF is benign or adverse is not always straightforward. Consider an example. Curt Hagquist and David Andrich (2017) used Swedish data from the Health Behaviour in School-Aged Children Psychosomatic Checklist (HBSC-SCL) to evaluate gender DIF. The checklist asks:

In the last six months, how often have you had the following complaints: headache, stomachache, backache, feeling low, irritability or bad tempered, feeling nervous, difficulties in getting to sleep, feeling dizzy.

They found gender DIF for stomachache in grade 9, with girls reporting problems to a higher extent than expected by the Rasch model. In another paper Hagquist (2019) defends the hypothesis that the gender DIF for stomachache is due to girls' menstruation.

The question is whether the gender DIF found in the stomachache question is benign or adverse. The answer to this question, Hagquist (2019, 8) argues, depends on whether we think complaints caused by "gender specific biological conditions should be a part of the measure of psychosomatic problems."[6] In other words, are complaints caused by menstruation relevant or irrelevant to the HBSC-SCL? If the question indicates benign DIF, then keeping it in the scale enhances validity and fairness, while maintaining invariance among the items (with some loss of model fit). If the question indicates adverse DIF, then deleting or resolving the question will enhance validity and fairness, but it will destroy the invariance of the item parameters among groups (Hagquist 2019).[7] If we make the wrong assignment, we risk the validity of the instrument and the fairness of its application. In other words, what I refer to as fit for purpose is at risk.

What should we take away from this example? One thought is that "psychosomatic" was not properly conceptualized in the context of the HBSC-SCL.[8] The reasoning goes something like this: if due diligence had been done during qualitative research—or, as I argue, epistemic dialogue—questions of relevance wouldn't (or would only rarely) arise. Certainly, in the previous decade, as the literature on patient-centered measures has emphasized the dearth of theoretical development, and the FDA (2009) has emphasized content validity, this thought seems to be common. When questions about the relevance of an item content occur, the answer is usually better questionnaire development. In other words, if proper consultation with patients, people with disabilities, and other ill persons in conjunction with clinicians and health researchers had occurred during the questionnaire's development phase, we wouldn't be in the position of wondering whether this DIF is benign or adverse.

This response reinforces the use and expectations of standardized questions. If epistemic dialogue can offer a sufficiently well-understood construct, then this knowledge will eliminate ambiguity in the meaning of the questions and answers posed in the measure. It's the ambiguity over the meaning of a positive answer to the stomachache question in the HBSC-SCL that causes the problem; that is, is it benign or adverse DIF? But can epistemic dialogue speak to underdetermination? I think this response is overly optimistic. Epistemic dialogue and well-conceptualized constructs are important and, indeed, necessary for the reasons I discussed in the previous chapter, but they are not sufficient to solve the problem of underdetermination. We are mistaken if we think there is some point in the future where questionnaire development renders respondent answers transparent to our interests. Rather, as I argue in the next section, questions of relevance will continue to affect patient-centered measures even if patients participate with researchers as epistemic equals in the developmental phase. This suggestion means standardized questions used in patient-centered measures will often fail to achieve mechanical objectivity in part because we aren't always sure in advance of asking questions what counts as irrelevant vis-à-vis the construct of interest. It also means that coordination of patient-centered measures with the constructs they seek to quantify is not one and done: patient-centered measures require ongoing coordination. I will discuss this point toward the end of the chapter.

4.2.3. Context Sensitivity and Response Shift

At least part of the reason why better questionnaire development is insufficient is that patient-centered constructs tend to be context and time sensitive. No matter how inclusive and rigorous we are at the development phase of patient-centered measures, we are likely to face questions of relevance as respondents answer questions during what we might call the "response phase," that is, the phase of patient-centered measures when they are no longer being developed, but rather being used. Context sensitivity can affect both longitudinal studies and cross-sectional studies. Consider cross-sectional studies first. The Covid-19 pandemic, climate change, innovations around health technologies, a greater awareness of period stigma, and more transparency around menstruation (United Nations Women 2019; United Nations 2022)—all have the potential to impact respondents' understanding of patient-centered constructs like quality of life and physical functioning. More specifically, regarding the question about stomachache pain from the HBSC-SCL, context sensitivity has the potential to impact what counts as a *complaint* about pain, as opposed to pain that is tolerated or concealed (The Lancet 2018). The understanding of quality of life, physical functioning, or a complaint that arises from events such as these may be different from what was intended (after conducting epistemic dialogue). Nonetheless, these differences don't necessarily render respondent understandings irrelevant. Indeed, it may render them better—*more* relevant. For instance, before the Covid pandemic many of us took face-to-face social interaction for granted or even wished for less of it. Arguably, face-to-face interactions were part of the background understanding of general subjective health, but it probably wasn't articulated in most cases. The pandemic, however, turned face-to-face interactions into something that many explicitly value as a part of their subjective health. It's likely that many now take face-to-face interactions into account when answering questions about general subjective health. The modalities of human interactions available to us are now part of what we must consider when conceptualizing general health; for most of us this was not the case prior to the pandemic.

At the same time, not all differences should be taken as improvements. Epistemic dialogue during questionnaire development has an important role, which shouldn't be undermined. But if epistemic dialogue informs but does not determine relevance, then how do we know when respondent answers are relevant or irrelevant to the construct of interest? The relevance and irrelevance of respondent understandings have been explored most extensively through the literature on response shift. Discussing response shift means turning our attention from context and time sensitivity in cross-sectional studies to longitudinal ones.

Differences between on-the-ground respondent understandings and those intended after epistemic dialogue don't automatically render respondents' answers irrelevant, because context can initiate legitimate changes. Similarly, in longitudinal studies, time can initiate changes in understanding between respondents' first encounter with a questionnaire and the second or third time they encounter it (which can be months later). Some unexpected changes may be relevant, others not. The unexpected changes considered relevant are referred to as response shift effects. This is the phenomenon I discussed in the introduction to this chapter. Response shift is defined as a change in the self-evaluation of a target construct. For instance, consider a question from the European Organisation for Research and Treatment of Cancer Quality of Life Questionnaire:

Were you limited in pursuing your hobbies or other leisure time activities?
Not at all
A little
Quite a bit
Very much

In Marjan Westerman et al.'s (2008) "think aloud" study, one patient answered this question in his first interview: "My hobby is working in the garden, that's very difficult." He chose as his answer "quite a bit." During the second interview, he said, "I'm reading at the moment. Gardening is not possible anymore." In this instance he chose, "a little." One way to think about response shift is in terms of priorities. From the first interview to the second, the man in this example changed what he valued doing in his leisure time. This in turn affected how he evaluated his limitations. It's a good example of response shift because it illustrates the puzzle response shift traditionally posed, namely, patient-reported quality of life can improve (from being limited "quite a bit" to "a little") while respondents can do less ("gardening is not possible anymore"). Early research on response shift focused on how to make sense of this apparent contradiction.

Response shift effects have been documented in a variety of settings and a wide range of diseases: cancer, stroke, coronary artery disease, different types of surgeries, diabetes, multiple sclerosis, back pain, and hearing loss (Vanier et al. 2018). Researchers studying response shift have argued for over two decades that it is relevant to our understanding of patient-centered measurement. There is now a broad consensus that response shift effects represent important information. Indeed, the possibility that subjective health outcomes can fly in the face of objective health assessments is the basis on which patient-centered measures were founded (Rapkin and Schwartz 2019). Response shift research helps us to understand and be more responsive to these kinds of differences. From this perspective response shift is not a side project within patient-centered measurement, but rather the soul of the discipline.

Nonetheless, within the consensus of response shift's importance, there is disagreement about what response shift *is* and how to model it (Rapkin and Schwartz 2019; Vanier et al. 2021), which in turn affects what respondent understandings count as relevant and irrelevant. There are two different interpretations of response shift. The first one theorizes response shift through a model of cognitive appraisal (Rapkin and Schwartz 2004; Schwartz and Rapkin 2004). The second one theorizes response shift through the principle of conditional independence (PCI) (Vanier et al. 2021). In what follows I consider both interpretations in an extended example. As I indicated in the introduction to this chapter, I focus my discussion on how these accounts interpret response shift as a theoretical phenomenon; I am less interested in their respective methodologies. I discuss the appraisal approach first.

4.2.3.1. Response Shift: The Appraisal Model

Bruce Rapkin and Carolyn Schwartz jointly developed the appraisal approach to response shift in 2004 (Rapkin and Schwartz 2004; Schwartz and Rapkin 2004). Their approach is unique in its attempt to (1) theorize response shift and (2) develop measures to quantify appraisal. Other approaches tend to lack both theoretical considerations of response shift and direct measurement. The appraisal approach, as the name suggests, begins not with response shift, but with appraisal. Appraisal is not specific to response shift. In fact, Rapkin and Schwartz (2004) argue that *any* response to a question in a patient-centered measure is a function of a four-part cognitive appraisal process. Accordingly, when respondents are asked to answer a question, they must first *induce a frame of reference* regarding relevant experiences, then within this frame of reference they must *sample specific experiences*, for example, their "worst moments" or "recent flare ups" (Rapkin et al. 2017). Each sampled experience is then judged against *a standard of comparison*, (e.g., compared to others my age, compared to my ability to function last year), and, finally, respondents combine their evaluation of relevant experiences *in an algorithm* to arrive at an answer (Rapkin and Schwartz 2004). Respondent answers are a function of appraisal because appraisal determines the meaning of the question for a respondent.

Response shifts are defined as changes in appraisal over time. Indeed, the appraisal approach is an extension of the Sprangers and Schwartz (1999) definition of response shift, which recognizes three manifestations: recalibration, reprioritization, and reconceptualization. Recalibration is a change in a respondent's internal standards of measurement; for example, what counts as severe pain before childbirth is plausibly different afterward. In the appraisal framework, recalibration is operationalized as a change in standards (Rapkin and Schwartz 2019). Reprioritization is a change in a respondent's values; for example, what I value doing in my leisure time may change over the course of a long illness, which may in turn affect how I evaluate my limitations. Reprioritization is operationalized in appraisal as a change in sampling or algorithm (Rapkin and Schwartz 2019). Reconceptualization is a change in the definition of the target construct; for example, I may understand good health as synonymous with daily cardiovascular exercise but come to understand it as a function of nutrition after a diagnosis of rheumatoid arthritis. Reconceptualization is taken to manifest as an appraisal change regarding frame of reference (Rapkin and Schwartz 2019).

Rapkin et al. (2017, 2018) have created multiple measures of appraisal, the Quality of Life Appraisal Profile (QOLAP), the QOLAPv2, and the Brief Appraisal Inventory (BAI). The QOLAP measures appraisal with eight open-ended questions focused on personal goals, concerns, and the meaning of quality of life. This measure requires coding on over 30 attributes, and thus significant time is required to work with it (Rapkin et al. 2017). The QOLAPv2 was designed as a more practical measure of appraisal requiring fewer resources. Instead of open-ended questions it offers 85 closed-end Likert-scaled questions and 12 orthogonal second-order component scores.

Consider, for instance, the questions posed in the QOLAPv2. Frame of reference is measured in two sections. One section of 16 questions focuses on "meaning of quality of life," where respondents are asked the extent to which their definition of quality of life agrees or disagrees with themes such as "having a healthy lifestyle" and "looking back on my legacy." In the second frame of reference section, respondents are asked 25 questions about their goals. They are asked to rate "how much like me" are statements such as, "There is much more I want to accomplish at my job" and "I am very concerned about growing as a religious or spiritual person." Sampling of experience is measured in the QOLAPv2 with 14 questions that ask respondents how often during the day's interviewing they have used criteria such as "worst moments" or "what your doctor has told you about your health" to respond to questions. From these 85 questions, second-order analysis yields 12 component scores: wellness focus, health worries, recent challenges, spiritual focus, relationship focus, maintain roles, independence, reduce responsibilities, pursue dreams, anticipating decline, worry-free, and lightness of being. These second-order component scores represent patterns of appraisal across the different domains; for example, the wellness focus represents a pattern across frame of reference (goals), experience sampling, and standards of comparison.

The third measure, the BAI, asks 23 Likert-scaled questions about how often (always to never) respondents thought about a specific appraisal approach, for instance, "maintaining a positive outlook, even when things are going badly," "being free from money problems," and "trying not to complain about your health to others." It was developed after analysis of themes and patterns of appraisal from both the QOLAP and QOLAPv2.

These appraisal measures have been used in modeling studies to examine and quantify response shift effects (Rapkin and Schwartz 2004; Schwartz et al. 2020). The appraisal measure is applied to the same population being measured on a patient-centered instrument. The idea is to capture, on the one hand, change in appraisal with, say, the QOLAPv2, and on the other hand, to isolate unexpected change in, say, quality of life, from the applications of the patient-centered measure. Health researchers refer to unexpected change as "residual variance." Unexpected change or "residual variance" is the difference between the observed value of change scores from applications of patient-centered measures and the change scores one would predict given the demographics, health, and intervention status of the respondents to the measure (Rapkin and Schwartz 2019). In other words, when respondents say their quality of life is better than it was last month but their health is worse, this is an unexpected change in quality of life (because we tend to assume health and quality of life go together). It is the kind of change we'd expected to see as part of the "residual variance" calculation. Once we have isolated the residual variance, the next step is to test whether changes in appraisal can explain the residual variance. Response shift is inferred only when changes in appraisal can explain residual variance; the variance it cannot explain is assumed to be error (Rapkin and Schwartz 2019, 2021).

The appraisal approach to response shift is significant for at least two reasons. It takes seriously that respondents' points of view are integral to the evaluation of patient-centered constructs (Schwartz and Rapkin 2004). This "seriousness" is reflected in the way cognitive change is problematized. Second, it responds to problems of identifying construct irrelevance. Recall above I suggested two problems with identifying construct irrelevance in patient-centered measures, a practical problem and a theoretical problem.

Practically, we cannot usually work backward from respondent answers to understand how questions are interpreted. Theoretically, the claim of model misfit is underdetermined by the evidence—it can reflect relevant or irrelevant changes in respondent understandings. Schwartz and Rapkin (2004) speak to both problems at once with their theory of appraisal. On the practical side, measures of appraisal provide insight into how questions are understood, which in turn help make respondent answers meaningful. As Schwartz and Rapkin (2004, 4) write,

> Differences in appraising QOL and attendant problems in discerning the meaning of QOL scores cannot simply be dismissed as measurement error, bias in perception or misuse of scales. The individual's particular vantage point is not arbitrary, it is intrinsic to rating of QOL. Unfortunately, in the usual case, QOL measurement does not preserve any information about the psychological process used to arrive a particular score. . . . There are many ways to arrive at a rating, but QOL ratings in and of themselves convey no "backstory" about the process of appraisal. Without this information, it is impossible to understand what a score means or how to validate it.

On the theoretical side, appraisal theory provides criteria for determining relevance. According to Rapkin and Schwartz (2019) a response shift requires three conditions.

1. A discrepancy between what is expected or predicted by the model and what is observed, for example, model misfit or lack of correlation.
2. A change in appraisal, that is, recalibration, reprioritization, or reconceptualization.
3. Changes in appraisal must be able to explain the unexpected observed change.

These conditions, particularly the latter two, provide a plausible solution to the underdetermination of evidence: changes that meet these conditions are relevant to the construct of interest.

4.2.3.2. Violation of the Principle of Conditional Independence
Frans Oort (2005) and subsequently Oort and colleagues (2009) developed a different approach to response shift. This approach takes the principle of conditional independence (PCI) as its point of departure. PCI is not

a difficult concept, but it's helpful to begin with independence and work up to conditional independence. Independence in probability says if I consider two events and I know one occurred, this knowledge has no effect on the outcome of the second event. People who study probability like to use coin flips as examples. If I flip a coin and it lands on heads, this outcome has no effect on the subsequent flip of the coin. Coin flips are independent events. Conditional independence refers to a situation where two events are independent of one another *given* a third event: A and B are conditionally independent of C if and only if given knowledge of C, knowledge of whether A occurs provides no information on the likelihood of B occurring, and knowledge of whether B occurs provides no information on the likelihood of A occurring. Think again about coin flips. The canonical example for conditional independence is a biased coin. Say you have a coin that is biased to land on heads 99% of the time. You flip it and it lands on heads; you flip it again and it lands on heads. Once you know you have a biased coin, each flip is independent of the other flips. In other words, knowing how the coin landed in the previous flip provides no further information about how the next flip will land given that you know the coin is biased. In the context of patient-centered measurement conditional independence is fulfilled if, given knowledge of, say, physical health, the scores on a test for functioning are invariant for, say, gender. Intuitively, this means, considering the physical health of our sample population, knowing their scores on the test tells us nothing about their gender, and knowing their gender tells us nothing about their scores.

In 1989 Gideon Mellenbergh introduced violations of PCI to define measurement bias. Consequently, in cases of measurement bias, test scores are not independent of variables such as gender, age, or disease. Following this introduction, Fran Oort (2005) and Visser et al. (2005) incorporated a range of measurement issues, including response shift, under the PCI umbrella. A violation of conditional independence indicates response shift when observed scores on repeated administrations of a test are not independent of the time of the test (or individual characteristics that change with time) given the true attribute values of respondents at the time of the test (Oort et al. 2009). Oort et al. (2009, 1130) write, "With response shift present, observed changes in respondents' test scores cannot be fully explained by true changes in the attribute that we want to measure."

In 2019 a group of international and interdisciplinary researchers convened in four working groups, each focusing on a different aspect of response shift. In the interest of transparency, I should say I was one of these researchers, although as will become clear, my ideas on response shift have evolved. The idea behind the meetings was to examine critically previous work done on response shift to summarize, clarify, and identify future research areas (Sprangers et al. 2021). My group was tasked with the definition and theoretical underpinnings of response shift. This group reinforced Oort et al.'s 2009 definition: response shift is a special case of violation of conditional independence; it occurs when observed change cannot be fully explained by target change at t_n.

On this account response shift is an effect of some cause, but the nature of the cause is left somewhat open-ended. Rather than theorize about the specific cause of response shift (as appraisal theory does), this account emphasizes an operational model and chains of causality. There are two chains of causality that can lead to a response shift. The first is the most common: (1) the impact of a catalyst (e.g., a health event or experience) on a person's interpretation of a questionnaire is mediated by a mechanism (e.g., psychological adaptation) or (2) there is a direct effect of a catalyst (e.g., shock of car accident) that influences a person's interpretation of a questionnaire when it is administered immediately after the event (Vanier et al. 2021).

The significance of the "PCI" account of response shift is best understood in comparison with the appraisal account. Both accounts begin roughly in the same place: with model misfit or lack of correlation. Thus, response shift begins with a discrepancy between expected and observed scores. But unlike the appraisal account, the PCI account more or less ends at the same place. The PCI account is part of the tradition of evidence-based medicine in turning away from mechanistic reasoning in favor of statistical reasoning (Guyatt et al. 1922). Statistical reasoning tends to "black-box" explanations of how and why something happens in favor of comparisons (Howick et al. 2010). Accordingly, the PCI account black-boxes explanations of how and why response shift occurs and simply compares observed scores with expected scores. Indeed, the point of Vanier et al.'s (2021) article is to make a distinction between what response shift *is* and how and why it occurs. As Vanier et al. (2021, 3316) write, "This more specific definition considers response shift as an effect but does not explain how this effect occurs." Later in the article different theories and approaches that might explain response shift are discussed, but the article is agnostic. Response shift may or may not be recalibration, reprioritization, or reconceptualization; changes in appraisal may or may not lead to response shift.

In addition to black-boxing the mechanism(s) responsible for response shift, the PCI approach, unlike the appraisal approach, defines response shift as measurement bias. Indeed, measurement bias is baked into the PCI definition of response shift. When managing measurement bias, researchers typically try to minimize and model it. Consider first how the PCI definition models response shift. Vanier et al. (2021) provide a visual model, which illustrates different cognitive pathways that can lead to measurement scores (Figure 4.1).

When the pathways illustrated in the model equal zero, then change in the target construct is fully explained by observed changes in the measure (no response shift). When the pathways are nonzero, there is a response shift effect. Response shift is thus modeled as the gap between expected and observed scores at t_2. The PCI model further identifies two nonzero pathways for response shift, a direct pathway and a more common mediated pathway (discussed above). We might define response shift on the PCI account thus:

1. A discrepancy between expected scores and observed scores over time in which observed change is not fully explained by target change
2. A discrepancy explained in terms of a direct or mediated pathway as described by Vanier et al. (2021)

Although I think this second condition could plausibly make the PCI account stronger, Vanier et al. (2021) don't make much of it. Instead, they emphasize a variety of response shift methods that examine discrepancies between expected change and observed change (Vanier et al. 2021). As a theory of response shift, this is a very thin account, and it ends much where I started my discussion of construct irrelevance: lack of correlation or model misfit, which leads to underdetermination. Indeed, at the end of the article, Vanier et al. (2021, 3319) gesture briefly at this underdetermination: "Violation of the PCI may be considered a necessary but not a sufficient condition for the occurrence of response shift," in which case "Alternative explanations need to be ruled out before the conclusion that response shift has occurred is warranted" (2021, 3320). They provide a table of these other explanations, for instance, response bias, framing effect, recall bias, and so on, but there is no discussion of how they would be ruled out.

As I've said, the PCI account treats response shift as measurement bias. Researchers usually try to minimize and model bias. Above I discuss how this account models response shift, but what about minimizing it? In my

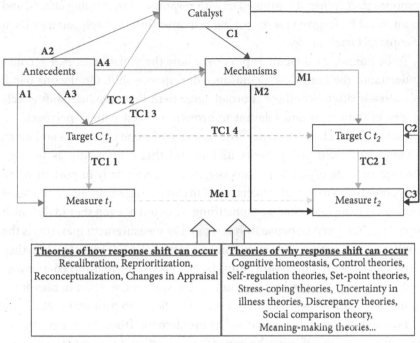

Notes: Target C = Target Construct. t_1 = first time. t_2 = second time.

Catalyst: An health event or life experience.

Antecedents: More or less stable characteristics of the persons (e.g., age, coping style, impairments) and their environment (i.e., the content in which individuals live).

Mechanisms: Behavioral, cognitive and affective processes individuals adopt to accommodate the catalyst.

Target construct: The construct that is being measured, e.g., quality of life.

Measure: Any evaluation-based self-report, e.g., patient-reported outcome measure.

All the paths are labels using a letter corresponding to their cause (e.g., A paths are coming from Antecedents, TC paths are coming from Target Construct)

Figure 4.1 PCI response shift model at two points in time: t_1 and t_2. Response shift is modeled as an effect that occurs from t_1 to t_2 through pathways M2 and C3. In pathways TC1$_4$ and Me1$_1$ the variability of the target construct and its measure is carried from time 1 to time 2, there is no response shift.

experience, response shift researchers are usually uneasy with this suggestion. Response shift is not conceptualized as a *mis*understanding, but rather a legitimate change in understanding. In fact, some clinical specialties such as rehabilitation medicine strive to evoke a response shift in patients. These kinds of considerations are what make response shift interesting and special. Yet when we attend to the PCI account, it's hard to see what is special about response shift. When it is lumped in with response bias, framing effects, and so on, you'd be forgiven for imagining response shift is simply another form of construct irrelevance.

To be honest, it's difficult to pin down how the violation of PCI account understands the normative significance of response shift. On the one hand, as I already discussed, there is broad agreement that response shift effects represent important and relevant information about patient perspectives. Vanier et al. (2021, 3310) write, "The *meaning* of some constructs and items is time dependent and patients understand them differently as they go through new life experiences. This suggestion is especially important when instruments aim to be patient-centered." In this passage, response shift effects don't seem to be understood as something we could or even should diminish or reduce. Yet when response shift is treated as measurement bias, this is the implication. This tension is overcome in Oort et al.'s 2009 article when they write that while response shift "must be accounted for to avoid contamination of measurement and explanation . . . the substantive effect of bias or response shift can be meaningful" or even "beneficial" to patients (1135). Here response shift is clearly understood as problematic from the perspective of measurement, even if from the patient's perspective it is good. This is kind of like saying, "It's OK if you believe your life is better now than it was three months ago—and we're glad for you that you think it is—but for the purposes of science we need to quantify your bias so it doesn't contaminate our measurement." Maybe this rendition is too harsh. But the PCI account can't avoid the fact that response shift is defined in contrast to true change. If the construct is quality of life, then it is difficult to see how response shift doesn't amount to saying people are wrong about their quality of life even if being wrong is beneficial for their mental health. I am not the only one to notice this problem. Rapkin and Schwartz (2021, 3360) write: "Both the Vanier et al. and Sawatzky et al. papers promote a perspective that response shift is a form of bias in measurement. This position is difficult to reconcile with an understanding of response shift as meaningful change."

I started this discussion of response shift because patient-centered constructs tend to be context and time sensitive. While lack of correlation or model fit may alert us to the possibility of construct irrelevance, this claim is often underdetermined by the evidence. Moreover, managing context and time sensitivities cannot be wholly dealt with during questionnaire development. I suggested if questions of relevance aren't solved during questionnaire development, then we must focus on the response phase of the questionnaire. I turned to the response shift literature to look for an example of how questions of relevance might be solved. In this literature we see a difference in interpretation: the appraisal approach and the PCI approach. While the appraisal approach provides a strategy for critically engaging with respondent understandings that are different from those anticipated, the PCI approach treats all differences in understanding alike; while the appraisal approach provides criteria for identifying response shift, the PCI approach seems ill-equipped to discriminate response shift from other forms of bias.

Recall I discussed two problems identifying construct irrelevance in patient-centered measures: a practical problem and a theoretical problem. The PCI account cannot overcome either of these. First, unlike the appraisal account, it doesn't provide insight into what respondents mean by their answers, and, second, it doesn't go beyond lack of correlation or model misfit in identifying construct irrelevance. The appraisal account, on the other hand, has an importance that extends beyond the debate over response shift; it is fertile. Response shift refers fundamentally to changes in the self-evaluation of a target construct over time, and it is one way patient-centered measures are context sensitive. But as I discussed earlier, relevant context sensitivity may also occur when respondents encounter the questionnaire for the first time, which I will refer to as response *initiation*. Appraisal measures provide insight into how respondents are interpreting questions through the use of, for instance, a frame of reference or standard of comparison. We can use these measures to conceptualize and identify relevant changes in understanding regarding response *shift*, but we might also use them to identify relevant changes in understanding regarding initiation. Relevant change, whether from response shift or response initiation, suggests that coordination between patient-centered measures and their construct(s) is ongoing. I'll have more to say about ongoing coordination in the next two sections.

4.3. Opportunity to Learn

Turning away from construct irrelevance, I now want to consider another concern the *Standards* raises regarding validity and fairness, namely, opportunity to learn. Recall that "the *Standards*" refers to *Standards for Education and Psychological Testing* (American Educational Research Association 2014), in which fairness is considered a fundamental validity issue. The *Standards* defines opportunity to learn as the extent to which test takers or respondents to questionnaires have been "exposed to the tested constructs through their educational program and/or have had exposure to or experience with the language or the majority culture required to understand the test" (American Educational Research Association 2014, 221). The idea is if respondents aren't familiar with the construct being assessed, then inferences about their ability level (for instance) may be invalid. When inferences lead to, say, diagnosis, promotion, or resources, then invalid inferences are also unfair inferences. Opportunity to learn is an important consideration for a measure's fitness for purpose.

Opportunity to learn is of particular relevance to *standardized* tests and questionnaires. Opportunity to learn is less relevant in the context of unstandardized questions since in this case the questions themselves offer the opportunity to learn. Recall my example from earlier when I asked what to do when my horse won't listen in lessons. In this case, I assumed my interlocutor understood my question as I intended it to be understood. Yet when the responses I received were unexpected, I had the opportunity to rethink my question and learn from the answers I received. That is how I came to understand my question differently: What should I do *in and out of the saddle as opposed to one or the other with respect to prevention* when Toni won't listen in lessons? Throughout the process of interpreting and reinterpreting my question and answers, I ended up learning more than I anticipated when I asked my original question.

Standardized questions, however, do not offer an "opportunity to learn." Respondents must instead come to a test or questionnaire having already learned. This model resembles standardized testing in education. Students go to school or university, where they are given the opportunity to learn content about a subject matter from an authority on it. The assumption is the authority knows the subject better than the students, and thus students should learn how to think about the subject matter from the authority. In the context of standardized testing, there is a subtle three-way alignment that must be in place for the spirit of "opportunity to learn" to be fulfilled. Teachers must have sufficient knowledge of the subject matter; the curriculum must present the subject matter in ways that anticipate test questions, and the test must reflect the curriculum as it is taught to students. "Opportunity to learn" is perhaps a more positive way of saying that teachers "teach to the test." In the context of standardized tests, fairness requires it.

Yet, when dealing with questionnaires such as patient-centered measures, "teaching to the test" isn't practical. In the case of patient-centered measures, the FDA's emphasis on content validity, which I discussed in Chapter 3, serves as a substitute. Recall that content validity aims to ensure that the construct and questions in patient-centered measures reflect the experience and language of the population for whom the measure is designed. The reason it aims to do this is to secure the inferences from respondent answers to the construct of interest. I argued in Chapter 3 that epistemic dialogue is necessary for the development of patient-centered measures: here I will argue, as I also did in the previous section, that this approach is not sufficient for validity or fairness.

It may go without saying at this point, but standardized questions are not used to learn something new about a subject matter. Instead, we use them to locate someone or some population within a subject matter, that is, within the construct or latent trait being measured.[9] For instance, when teachers ask standardized questions about the perimeter of geometric shapes, they are likely using them to locate students' ability levels vis-á-vis basic geometry. Similarly, when health researchers ask questions about subjective health status on the NHP, they want to locate patients within a landscape of good and poor subjective health status. Logically speaking, to locate someone or a population within a construct, we need to have some knowledge of the construct in advance of developing the test. We need to know, for instance, what good and poor subjective health status looks like, what exceptional and average math ability looks like.

Having knowledge of a construct in advance of developing a test is what makes it possible to ask standardized questions. When we ask standardized questions, we narrow a question's possibilities. Gone is the extensive array of contrast classes and relevance relations that usually characterize a question's potential. Gone too is the indeterminant nature of the questions' topic. Instead, we narrow what counts as the answer and what counts as the correct interpretation of the question. When we narrow the meaning of questions and answers, we also narrow the topic to which the questions refer. This narrowing requires some assumptions. We assume, for instance, that the question's topic—the construct we wish to measure—can and should be so narrowed. We also assume the questions and answers are understood similarly by those involved—teachers, researchers, students, and respondents. These two assumptions are related. Questions and answers stand in relation to a topic of interest. We ask questions and seek answers *about something*. This is a three-way relationship: questions, answers, and a subject matter or topic of interest. When we narrow the meaning of questions and answers, we also narrow the topic of the questions and answers. This narrowing is what makes "opportunity to learn" possible; we can teach to the test because we've narrowed down what it is important to know about a particular topic.

Philosophers have pointed out that narrowing down a topic—or as Sophia Efstathiou (2012, 2016) refers to it, founding a concept—is part of measurement. Founding is necessary because as Bradburn et al. (2017) argue, concepts in the medical and social sciences are often *Ballung* concepts. By this they mean that concepts like subjective health status and quality of life are vague and imprecise. In the natural habitat of everyday discourse quality of life can mean many things to many people. But if we want to use *Ballung* concepts scientifically—if we wish to measure them—then they must be "founded" (Efstathiou 2012, 2016). In other words, these everyday concepts must be "transfigured" into more precise, narrower ones (Efstathiou 2016). In founding a concept such as quality of life, we should be prepared, as Nancy Cartwright (2020, 279) says, "for both multiplication of concepts and loss of meaning." In other words, we should not be surprised when measures of quality of life proliferate with different operationalizations of the concept; nor should we be surprised that when measuring these constructs, we must sacrifice some of the meanings people give to it. This, they seem to suggest, is the price of measurement.

This picture of founded concepts motivates "opportunity to learn." If a measurement construct loses its everyday meaning in measurement, then all the more reason for respondents to have the opportunity to learn how it's operationalized before taking a test; all the more reason for people with disabilities, patients, and other ill persons to act as partners in the development of patient-centered measures. Indeed, it becomes clearer why fairness requires opportunity to learn in contexts where *Ballung* concepts are founded for scientific use. For surely it isn't fair for respondents to be assigned a place within a construct such as quality of life if the construct is likely to be used in an unfamiliar or unusual way.

When we combine founded *Ballung* concepts with the standardized questions in a measure or questionnaire, much of the validity and fairness rests on founding the *Ballung* concept appropriately for the purposes of the measure, and then teaching respondents how to understand it. In the case of patient-centered measures, founding the *Ballung* concept appropriately for the purposes of the measure must at the same time take into account what is meaningful to people with disabilities, patients, and other ill persons. This is the process of epistemic dialogue. We can now think of the outcomes of epistemic dialogue as founded concepts. Founded concepts are important and necessary for the development of patient-centered measures, but they cannot bear the weight of validity and fairness alone.

The *Standards'* "opportunity to learn" helps orient us to the role respondents' understanding plays in validity and fairness; namely, we need good reasons to believe respondents will understand the test or questionnaire as it is intended to be understood. But once we recognize this role, it's clear that we often don't have these good reasons. Moreover, as I discussed above, when respondents understand differently, their understandings are not always *mis*understandings. The understanding researchers and people with disabilities, patients, and other ill persons arrive at to operationalize a measure's construct during the development phase of measurement might be unfit for the particular population being measured during the response phase. The reasons for this are various: the population under measurement might be relevantly different from those who participated in developing the measure despite efforts to keep them the same; important aspects of the construct may have been overlooked in development despite efforts to unearth them; shared understandings are often new understandings, and they may fail to resonate with some or most of the population being measured, and, as I discussed above, patient-centered constructs are context and time sensitive. Thus, the time between questionnaire development and response initiation may alter how the population understands the questions, for example, a pandemic or changes in health technology.

Just as the picture of founded *Ballung* concepts helps make clear the rationale behind "opportunity to learn," it also alerts us to the tension between founded patient-centered concepts and opportunity to learn when "teaching to the test" is not practical. In the context of patient-centered measures, Bradburn et al. (2017) are correct: founding what are often *Ballung* concepts is necessary. But to ensure validity and fairness, we can't simply found these concepts and never look back. We cannot black-box measurement. Instead, patient-centered measures require ongoing coordination: to ensure respondents are understanding questions correctly, to ensure *researchers* are understanding questions correctly, and for the instruments and its models to be adjusted as needed.

As I discussed at the end of the previous section, appraisal measures may be a fruitful tool for the kind of ongoing assessment I have in mind. To be sure, appraisal measures were developed to assess the presence of response shift. When used in the service of inferring response shift, these efforts are geared toward detecting changes over time that culminate in recalibration, reprioritization, and reconceptualization. But appraisal need not be limited to response shift. At the heart of appraisal is the desire to contextualize standardized questions. Efforts at appraisal in patient-centered measures are philosophically reminiscent of van Fraassen's (1980) pragmatic explanation.[10] The relevance of this point, however, goes beyond a narrow interest in explanation (van Fraassen) or response shift (Rapkin and Schwartz). Indeed, as I've suggested here, it may be extended to include response initiation. When respondents answer questions for the first time, they may understand those questions differently than researchers intended, yet these differences may not be misunderstandings. The trick will be to develop criteria, as Rapkin and Schwartz have done with response shift, that help separate out *mis*understanding from different understanding.

4.4. Ongoing Coordination

Fitness for purpose requires the ongoing assessment of patient-centered measures; assessment that attends to respondents' answers and how they interpret the questions in these measures. This ongoing assessment is a form of coordination and re-coordination of measuring instruments with the constructs they aim to measure. Coordination in measurement is ongoing. It is also, as I discussed in Chapter 1, a hermeneutic process. This point is not specific to patient-centered measures or the social sciences more generally. Indeed, it is not specific to "self-interpreting animals," as Charles Taylor (1985) refers to us. No, this is a fact about measuring instruments at large. To see this point, consider Eran Tal's (2011) discussion of atomic clocks. On his account, one of the features of standardization projects is their ongoing nature. This point has not received as much attention as other aspects of Tal's work, so it's worth taking a closer look at what he says.

Duration, like temperature and psychological constructs such as physical functioning and quality of life, is not observable. When we conceptualize duration, our concepts are necessarily abstract and ideal. For instance, the "second" is defined by taking the fixed numerical value of cesium frequency Δv_{Cs}, the unperturbed ground-state hyperfine transition frequency of the cesium 133 atom, to be 1,192,631,770 when expressed in the unit Hz (BIPM 2019). No actual cesium atom ever satisfies this definition, nor do we have a complete understanding of what it would take to satisfy it. What we do have are atomic clocks, or more accurately cesium fountains, known as "primary standards." These instruments serve as a concrete model for the abstract and ideal definition of a second. There are 15 primary standards around the world used as primary realizations of the second. In these standards, cesium atoms are funneled down a tube where they pass through microwaves. During this process the atoms' electrons move between two specific energy levels. The frequency of the radiation released when the electrons transition can be used as the basis of duration (similar to the swinging of a pendulum).

These atoms, as with anything we try to measure, are subject to forms of uncertainty and bias. To "realize" the referent of the second (or come as close to it as we can), metrologists model primary clocks according to the individual uncertainties and biases that affect them. Accordingly, metrologists identify ways that the cesium fountains diverge from the theoretical ideal. The example that Tal (2011) provides is gravitational redshift. The definition of the standard second assumes cesium is in a flat space-time, that is, has the gravitational potential of zero. Cesium fountains, however, exist on earth, where the gravitational potential is greater than zero. General relativity theory predicts the cesium frequency will be red-shifted depending on the altitude of the laboratory where the primary standard is located. Redshifts thus indicate measurement bias. The de-idealization process provides a magnitude for the predicted redshift; this correction plus an estimate of uncertainty is added to the cesium fountain's outcome. This de-idealization process is considered adequate when two conditions of what Tal (2011) refers to as the "Robustness Condition" are met: (1) the outcomes of a cesium clock converge on the outcomes from the other cesium clocks within the uncertainties ascribed to each clock and (2) the ascribed uncertainties are derived from appropriate theoretical and statistical models of each realization (Tal 2011, 1091).

This example has been used throughout the philosophy of measurement literature to highlight coordination (Tal 2011), calibration (Tal 2017), and the application of robustness in measurement (Basso 2017). But Tal's work also has another lesson: the standardization of time is an ongoing project (Tal 2016).[11] Coordination cannot be done a single time. This isn't to say robustness conditions are never met, but rather robustness requires continual assessment and maintenance. Another way to put this same point is to say that as metrologists strive for more accurate clocks, they must continue to coordinate units of time with their measuring instruments. This coordination can take the shape of modeling uncertainties in greater detail, modeling new uncertainties, adjusting, and maintaining the measuring instrument or even redefining the unit definition. This is the work of metrology. It is an ongoing dialogue among the unit definition, cesium clocks, and statistical models; it is an ongoing project of fitting part to whole. This is also the work of patient-centered measurement: an ongoing dialogue among questionnaires, constructs, people with disabilities, patients, and other ill persons, respondents, researchers, and models.

4.5. Conclusion

The ongoing coordination I argue for requires a reconceptualization and reframing of patient-centered measures. I suggest we think of these instruments as requiring a similar kind of ongoing coordination as clocks. Appraisal measures may play an important role in coordinating patient-centered measures by helping us stay attuned and nimble in the face of patients' points of view by helping us identify relevant dimensions of the constructs we measure. Information from appraisal measures may feed into coordination in different ways. For instance, we might use appraisal information to adjust our interpretation of measurement outcomes for some subpopulation. We might think of this adjustment as similar to the way uncertainty budgets work with cesium fountains (with the important caveat that this information is not bias). We might alter patient-centered measures themselves to better reflect respondent understandings (or avoid them) or we might redefine the construct of interest—perhaps splitting it into two constructs or reconceptualizing it altogether.

Reframing patient-centered measures as requiring ongoing coordination means reconceptualizing the roles that invariance and standardization play in these measures. We need to stop thinking of invariance as a property of constructs but rather as an artifact of measurement. We maintain the appearance of invariance over time and populations because we rely on, for example, appraisal information to contextualize respondent answers and thus measurement outcomes. Similarly with standardization. Standardization as mechanical objectivity isn't a realistic or desirable practice in patient-centered measures. It isn't realistic because respondents continue to understand questions differently than researchers intend. It isn't desirable because patient-centered measures are context sensitive. We need to shift to understand standardization as a limited but practical tool. For instance, standardizing the wording of questions simplifies questionnaires and may limit the burden on respondents and researchers. But standardizing the wording of questions does not standardize their meaning—nor should we intend it to. After epistemic dialogue with researchers, people with disabilities, patients, and other ill persons, we may be confident and justified in believing a particular set of questions is the right ones to ask. In other words, we might be confident that we understand the geography of the construct well enough to pose a question with standardized wording and response options. But because patient-centered measures aim to capture patient perspectives and because we know time can alter what is relevant to a construct, we must acknowledge that the questions posed lack interpretive precision. This is a feature, not a glitch.

In the next chapter I will continue to work out some of these implications for my proposal of ongoing coordination for patient-centered measures. In doing so I turn my attention to a set of issues, which I refer to broadly as the measurability of patient-centered constructs. When response shift researchers talk about the relevance of patient perspectives on, say, quality of life, they make a subtle and unexplored distinction between the construct and the perspectives respondents have on it. These perspectives, they seem to say, are relevant to understanding quality of life but are not themselves part of quality of life. This distinction is maintained in Rapkin and Schwartz's appraisal theory: appraisal measures and quality of life measures are different measures of different phenomena. One measures perspectives on quality of life, and the other measures quality of life. In the next chapter I will discuss this distinction. I'll also examine how this distinction holds up against the backdrop of recent philosophical discussions of the measurability of well-being and quality of life, as well as what measurability amounts to on my own account.

PART III
ADDRESSING CONCERNS

5

Are Patient-Centered Constructs Measurable?

In Chapters 3 and 4 I developed an epistemic theory for patient-centered measures. This theory does not attempt to theorize the constructs patient-centered measures assess, constructs such as quality of life and physical functioning. Rather it provides a procedural account of patient-centered measures, which is centered around two requirements:

1. Epistemic dialogue
2. Ongoing coordination

In Chapter 3 I discussed how people with disabilities, patients, and other ill persons should play a role in the development of patient-centered measures. Specifically, I argued they should participate as equals with health researchers in epistemic dialogue. In Chapter 4 I turned from the role people with disabilities, patients, and other ill persons play in developing these measures to the role they play as respondents. I argued that validity and fairness, what I call fitness for purpose, requires ongoing coordination of constructs with patient-centered measures. Because patient-centered measures are context and time sensitive, we cannot assume the intended meaning of the questions and answers will remain appropriate from measure development through to its many applications. Changes in meaning may occur during response initiation or through response shifts, and I suggested the appraisal approach, developed as an answer to response shift, may illuminate relevant changes in meaning.

Toward the end of Chapter 4, I suggested we think of invariance and standardization differently. Rather than think of invariance as a property of constructs, we should think of it as an artifact of measurement; rather than think of standardization as securing objectivity and fairness by "moving nature to the page" (Daston and Galison 2010, 120), we should think of it as a limited but practical tool. The idea here is that while patient-centered

Patient-Centered Measurement. Leah M. McClimans, Oxford University Press. © Oxford University Press 2024.
DOI: 10.1093/oso/9780197572078.003.0006

measures are developed using standardized questions, their use doesn't follow from a noninvariant construct. The use of standardized questions is practical and expedient. To the degree that patient-centered measures assume a noninvariant construct, this does not necessarily reflect their metaphysical reality, but often the transfiguration of *Ballung* concepts into founded constructs (Bradburn et al. 2017; Efstathiou 2016). Invariance and standardization thus understood are practical tools for patient-centered measurement, but, as I argued, without something like the use of appraisal adjuncts, the outcomes from these measures aren't fit for purpose. Appraisal adjuncts, I argued, could be used to correct course by providing contextual information that informs the interpretation of outcomes regarding, for instance, different subpopulations, new applications of a measure, and so on. Over time this information could feed into revisions of questions in a measure or even the development of new measures.

On my account of patient-centered measures, patient-centered constructs are time and context sensitive. To be sure, once they are founded we provisionally treat them as if they were invariant, but as we apply patient-centered measures to different populations or the same populations over time, we should anticipate variance. When this variance conforms to, for example, a response shift, then it is relevant and should be taken into account. Thus understood, patient-centered constructs are both time and context sensitive, and subject to measurement. In this chapter, I explore how this position compares to others.

The issue I want to explore in this chapter is measurability. To be sure, measurability means different things to different people—even within measurement—and there is ongoing debate about what is and is not measurable (e.g., Kyngdon 2008a, 2008b; Borsboom and Scholten 2008; Michell 2008). I touched on one way of thinking about measurability in Chapter 2 during my discussion of scale development and Rasch measurement theory. In this chapter, however, I am not concerned with scale types and whether interval-level representation is justified; rather I'm interested in the meaning and use of patient-centered constructs (Tal 2020) such as quality of life or physical functioning. In particular, I'm interested in how these terms are conceptualized and the consequences such conceptualizations have for an evaluation of their measurability.

In the well-being literature, philosophers tend to think of measurability in terms of *heterogeneity* (Hausman 2015; Alexandrova 2017). In this chapter I will share this interest. Heterogeneity is the idea that the goods required to make one individual's life go well are sufficiently different from those required to make other's lives go well. If the goods required for a good life are different for individuals, then measuring a good life is difficult. When you combine heterogeneity with a desire to create measures that are sensitive to individual perspectives, some philosophers of well-being conclude that these constructs aren't measurable, or if they are measurable, it's only in a limited way.

In this chapter I compare different accounts of heterogeneity: Dan Hausman's (2015) account in *Valuing Health: Well-Being, Freedom, and Suffering*, Anna Alexandrova's (2017) account in *A Philosophy for the Science of Well-Being*, and Bruce Rapkin, Caroline Schwartz, and colleagues' account across a number of papers. I argue that all three of these accounts conceptualize heterogeneity as an obstacle to measurement; that is, if we are able to measure well-being or quality of life, it's despite heterogeneity. For instance, Hausman and Alexandrova agree that constructs like well-being and quality of life are heterogeneous. For the purposes of using these measures to direct policy, Hausman thinks they are too heterogeneous; Alexandrova disagrees. She argues that if we focus on disease- and condition-specific measures, which she calls contextual well-being, then we can eliminate much of the heterogeneity that makes them problematic. Schwartz et al. (2020), on the other hand, locate heterogeneity not in patient-centered constructs, but in the perspectives of respondents. If this distinction makes sense (and I argue that it doesn't), it has the benefit of keeping patient-centered constructs homogenous.

Contrary to these approaches, I argue if we can measure patient-centered constructs at all it's because of heterogeneity, not despite it. In making this argument I help myself to some lessons from the philosopher Hans-Georg Gadamer's writings on hermeneutics. The upshot of these lessons is that while it's possible to talk abstractly about "constructs" and "subjective perspectives," it's only through the application of perspective to constructs that we have something we can meaningfully study, investigate, probe, or *measure*. In other words, it is only when respondents answer questions about patient-centered constructs that we have empirical content at all. The price of having patient-centered content that we can investigate and measure is that it comes to us as heterogeneous material because respondents will often answer questions differently from one another and differently over time. But, of course, I don't think this is much of a price because (1) patient-centered measures are an important force for good and (2) we can manage heterogeneity with creative applications of appraisal metrics and ongoing coordination.

5.1. Two Philosophies

Anna Alexandrova (2017) and Dan Hausman (2015) agree that generic well-being is too heterogeneous to measure for most health policy concerns. Before I say more about their arguments, a note on the use of "well-being." In the previous chapters I haven't been concerned with well-being. I've instead referred to "quality of life" or "physical functioning" as examples of patient-centered constructs. This said, I agree with Alexandrova (2017) when she argues that measures of quality of life and physical functioning (among many other kinds of measures) are implicitly about well-being. This is similar to Hausman's point (following on from Tim Scanlon (1998) that well-being is an "inclusive good." On this way of thinking, well-being isn't a good among other goods; it isn't the case that we have well-being, physical functioning, and mobility. Rather, "well-being" is the term we use to analyze or summarize, for example, the goods of physical functioning and mobility. Indeed, we might think of "quality of life" in the context of patient-centered measures as a synonym for well-being.[1] In any case, the point is I take Hausman's and Alexandrova's arguments on well-being to bear on patient-centered constructs; their arguments about the heterogeneity of well-being are thus relevant to my concerns in this book.

In *Valuing Health* (2015) Hausman is interested, primarily, in how health economists measure health. This orientation, which is common among philosophers interested in well-being, deserves an introduction since it has not been my primary topic of concern and it shapes Hausman's discussion. Hausman (2015, 28) argues early on that when health economists measure health, they don't develop measures that assess quantities of health directly; rather, they develop measures that assess the impact health has on what people care about. These measures aim to provide values for different health states. For many health economists we get these health *values* by measuring the impact a particular health state has on well-being or quality of life. So from this health economics perspective, the point of measuring well-being or quality of life is to get the health value of a certain health state. To relate Hausman's discussion to the content in this book, consider the EQ-5D.

The EQ-5D is a five-question, five-dimension, patient-centered utility measure. It asks respondents about mobility, self-care, usual activities, pain/discomfort, and anxiety/depression (Devlin and Brooks 2017). Each question has three possible answers. Five questions with three possible answers yields a total of 243 possible measurement indications or "health states" for the EQ-5D. During the development of the EQ-5D, researchers sought to "value" each of these health states by determining their impact on health-related quality of life. These valuations, which were obtained separately from the EQ-5D, serve as the interpretive key to the meaning of respondents' answers on the EQ-5D, that is, the meaning of the 243 possible indications. Thus, the EQ-5D doesn't measure quality of life so much as it picks out health states. These health states are then correlated with the value of these states.

How do health economists acquire the health values for these 243 health states? To find some of these valuations, researchers use the public's ranking of different health states using time trade-off (TTO) methods (Devlin and Brooks 2017). The TTO technique provides individuals with two scenarios, and they are asked which scenario they prefer. The length of time in the second scenario is varied until the individual is indifferent between the two. Traditionally the first scenario offers a chronic condition, i, that lasts for 10 years, followed by death. The second scenario offers full health for $xi <$ 10 years, followed by death. When the value of x is such that an individual is indifferent between the two scenarios, then the utility value for i is given by x / 10. An example of the TTO method could go something like this. Imagine you have chronic obstructive pulmonary disease (COPD). Now contemplate two scenarios. In one, you live 10 years with COPD without your health improving or deteriorating, and then you die. In another, you live less than ten years, but in perfect health, and then you die. The TTO method wants to know how much perfect health is as good as ten years with COPD. Say the answer we get from the public is six years. Then according to the TTO method, the utility value for COPD is .6; COPD has 60% the utility of being in perfect health.

Once researchers have enough of these direct preference elicitations from the public, the remainder of the health values are calculated using a utility function (Hausman 2015, 50). It is these valuations that are measures of quality of life, not the outcomes from the EQ-5D itself. Notice this process of valuing health closes the hermeneutic circle by answering the question "What is X?" with preference elicitation and "What is a good measure of X?" with TTO methods. This solution to the hermeneutic circle forestalls ongoing coordination of the sort I argued for in the previous chapter. At the same time, it also undermines inclusivity. But Hausman's beef with preference elicitation lies in a different direction.

Much of Hausman's book is taken up with how we should value health. TTO methods are one way to do it. This approach, as we saw, focuses on eliciting preferences from the public. The alternative to preference elicitation is to obtain health state valuations through measures of subjective well-being (by asking respondents questions about life satisfaction and positive and negative affect; see Chapter 1 for more on measures of subjective well-being). Both the TTO and subjective well-being approaches assume that health should be valued through its impact on well-being, but Hausman argues this reliance is problematic. Hausman's argument is complex, and not all the reasons he marshals against these measures are relevant to my purposes here, but at least one of them is. Hausman contends that TTO methods and subjective well-being measures fail because neither can measure with any precision the impact health has on well-being. This is because Hausman argues, well-being is too heterogeneous for health policy contexts.

Hausman's argument focuses on interpersonal heterogeny. When we think of well-being as a summary of an individual's well-being—an inclusive good—he argues there is nearly an infinite variety of goods that can justify a claim of positive well-being. For some its quiet nights reading; for others, it's pub crawls and discos. As Hausman (2015, 125) puts the point, "Everything from mascara to mussels, muscles, morality and Marxism may be good for one person or another." Part of the difficulty is that well-being, Hausman argues, is dependent on one's goals and values. Thus, one set of goods can appear to boost well-being, while the same set can undermine it when relative to different goals and values.

The problem heterogeny poses for measurement is how to rank these various sets of goods on a scale. What basis do we have for judging one set of goods as better than another set? What kind of life is better: one spent in quiet nights at home, or one spent in the pub or disco? To rank these goods, he argues we need a theory of well-being that explains what makes one set of goods better than another. Yet, according to Hausman, we either lack theories that do the job or we lack theories that do it with sufficient detail to be useful for the allocation of health resources. It's beyond my purposes here to provide a survey of Hausman's arguments against preference elicitation and subjective well-being, and, moreover, Alexandrova (2017, 109–15) has already done it. Suffice it to say he argues that these approaches paper over rather than solve the problem heterogeneity poses for measurement.

On the other hand, Hausman argues (2015, 131) measuring well-being is possible in a limited sort of way if we conceptualize well-being as flourishing. Hausman follows Richard Kraut in understanding flourishing as "the dynamic coherent integration of objective goods into an identity" (Hausman 2015, 141). If I prefer to live a transcontinental life because it makes certain objective goods (professional achievement, family stability, pleasure) possible in the context of my identity as a philosopher, wife, mother, and horseback rider, then this preference might indicate well-being (as opposed to insanity—as many have suggested). But it only is so indicative if I am evaluatively competent, rational, self-interested, well-informed, and have complete and transitive preferences among all my alternatives (Hausman 2015, 132). If these conditions are met *and* we have instruments that can track these preferences, then comparisons and even measurement of well-being are possible. When these conditions aren't met—and often they aren't—then comparisons of flourishing can still be made from a third-person perspective by "investigating the character, structure and activities of an agent" (Hausman 2015, 141). Nonetheless, confidence in these comparisons must be rather weak unless the differences among well-being are stark.

Despite endemic heterogeny, for Hausman it's *technically* possible to value health through its impact on well-being-as-flourishing. But this technical possibility doesn't amount to much in practice. Given its limitations, when and where these comparisons can be made won't always or even often line up with when and where we need them for the purposes of resource allocation. As Alexandrova (2017, 111) writes, "Hard cases abound." So, in the end, for the practical purposes of health policy, heterogeny is an obstacle to measuring generic well-being. Or, at least, so says Hausman. Alexandrova (2017, 116–17) eventually agrees: generic well-being cannot be measured for policy purposes. But even still, she wonders if we don't have more in common than Hausman suggests.

To be sure, well-being can be different things to different people. Yet among all the variety is there not a subset of goods we might agree is necessary to a good life? Alexandrova suggests there probably is. She turns to what she calls "Haybron-happiness" (Alexandrova 2015, 115). Haybron-happiness refers to Dan Haybron's (2008) conception of happiness, which amounts to feeling at home in oneself and the world, being engaged, and endorsing one's life. Even if a hip replacement is high on my list of priorities because I want a better seat in the saddle and it's low on yours because you can't take time off your feet, we both need some Haybron-happiness to get us through the day. On this view Haybron-happiness is a necessary but not sufficient condition of well-being, and drawing attention to it seems to undermine some of Hausman's heterogeny concern. If this assessment is correct, then Haybron-happiness—to the degree we can measure it—could be a decent proxy measure for generic well-being.

But can Haybron-happiness, as a proxy for well-being, guide health policy? Recall the point of this discussion is to value health through its impact on well-being. Does Haybron-happiness help us to value health? Are people with more Haybron-happiness in some relevant sense healthier? Perhaps they are mentally healthier, but if we want our metric to guide decisions about hip replacements and mole removals, Haybron-happiness might not cut it. Haybron-happiness is a kind of aspirational good. That is, we strive to be at home with ourselves and the world; we endeavor to remain engaged no matter what life throws at us, and if successful, many will endorse such a life. But then couldn't Haybron-happiness be conceived as a confounder rather than an indicator of health's value? Aiming for Haybron-happiness, my torn and worn labrum becomes a part of me, a part to which I strive to adjust. If I'm successful, I might be happier, but am I healthier? Am I less needful of a hip replacement? I'm not sure, but whatever I am, it's complicated.

For her part Alexandrova also isn't sure Haybron-happiness or complimentary measures are up to the task of measuring generic well-being, and her concern isn't very different from mine. Alexandrova is concerned about policy robustness. Say we can measure generic well-being. Whether these generic measures focus on something like Haybron-happiness or try to characterize a set of goods for individuals into an index, how well the outcomes translate into policy directives is unclear. Closing emergency departments in rural locations negatively affects the well-being of residents—in time, money, inconvenience spent traveling to urban hospitals, and loss of local revenue. But clinicians and policymakers often argue that patients are safer in bigger, better-equipped hospitals and that low-volume hospitals are inefficient.[2] How do we weigh up these different bundles of goods? On the one hand we have what we might call "the importance of community"; on the other we have "the importance of expertise and centralization." Even if we can measure generic well-being, how much more well-being must one bundle have over the other to justify a policy that will inevitably disadvantage some? Here again, whatever the proposed answer might be, it's complicated, and Alexandrova reckons it's *too* complicated. In that case, perhaps we're better off agreeing with Hausman: heterogeny is a measurement problem for generic well-being.

But generic well-being isn't the only option when we measure well-being. We can also measure condition and population-specific well-being, what Alexandrova (2017, 117–19) refers to as contextual well-being. Contextual well-being is "predicated of a particular kind of people in a specific type of circumstance" (Alexandrova 2017, 117). "Context specific" measures such as these abound in the patient-centered literature. Here are some examples: thyroid-specific patient-reported outcome measure (Watt et al. 2009); lupus patient-reported outcome in the Philippines (Navarra et al. 2013); and outcome measures for vascular malformations (Lokhorst et al. 2021). But how do disease- and population-specific measures solve the heterogeneity problem? Alexandrova supposes if we focus on kinds of people facing the same kinds of difficulties or conditions, then the sorts of goods that matter to them will be similar. The problem with Hausman's conception of well-being on her view is that it's too all-encompassing. When we think of well-being writ large—generic well-being—then it's not surprising we find significant heterogeny. People are different in the same circumstances, and people in different circumstances are even more different. But Alexandrova suspects we can find robust similarities among kinds of people if we cut the deck of goods in the right way. The difficulty with measuring generic well-being is the good we tend to share is too thin to justify health policy; our differences overwhelm it in ways that make health policy decisions sufficiently complicated to question the usefulness of the metric. But if we circumscribe the kind of well-being we're after, then perhaps they can do the policy jobs we ask of them.

To be sure, Alexandrova recognizes we'll have to generalize what makes for disease-specific well-being. Even when we cut the deck to measure the well-being of those with vascular malformations or lupus, the exact set of goods for each individual of this kind will differ. But if we focus on their kind and not their individuality—that is, if we focus on what makes them similar instead of what makes them different—we might get a set of goods to which the kind values similarly. Again, individuals subsumed under a kind may recognize some of these goods more than others, and for some there may be goods that do not apply. This might mean there are limits to the precision and responsiveness that some measures of well-being can achieve, but it doesn't undermine their measurement.

5.1.1. Putting Contextual Well-Being to the Test

One of the many aspects I appreciate in Alexandrova's work is her close consideration of well-being science. Like the best, her work is no pie-in-the-sky philosophy. So, in this spirit, I'd like to explore her suggestion that condition-specific—or in her words "contextual"—well-being is more measurable than generic well-being. I'd like to do this by examining an article in the literature on response shift that compares different measures' sensitivity to response shift affects.[3] In "Does Response Shift Impact Interpretation of Change Even among Scales Developed Using Item Response Theory?" Schwartz and colleagues (2020b) ask whether measures are differently sensitive to response shift depending on how the measure is developed. When characterizing measure development, the article combines mathematical measurement models with a consideration of construct terms. The article wonders if single-dimension measures developed in conjunction with item response theory (IRT) models are less sensitive to response shift effects than multidimension IRT models and CTT measures. We might understand this article as operationalizing and testing Alexandrova's proposal that contextual well-being is less sensitive to heterogeneity than generic well-being.

Consider how unidimensional IRT measures might constitute an operationalization of contextual well-being. IRT criteria for question selection is more restrictive than CTT, but not as restrictive as Rasch. IRT's restrictions come into play through its emphasis on construct unidimensionality and internal consistency. IRT methods thus narrow how much of a construct is represented by a measure. Consequently, IRT measures tend to be condition—or context—specific. For instance, in this article the IRT measures used come from the suite of Quality of Life in Neurological Disorders (NeuroQol) measures. Specifically, the authors use short forms of both applied cognition measures: one for general concerns and one for executive functions. They also use the NeuroQol Positive Affect and Well-Being (NeuroQol PAW) measure. This suite of NeuroQol instruments measure the mental and social effects of adults and children living with neurological conditions. By Alexandrova's lights, these are context-specific measures.

In the article by Schwartz et al. (2020b), these context-specific measures are compared to two sets of increasingly generic measures of well-being, that is, measures developed with multidimension IRT methods (which retain restrictive question selection criteria but increase construct representation through their multidimensionality) and CTT, which, as I discussed in

Chapter 1, is at the permissive end of the measurement models. In their study the multidimensional IRT methods are represented by the Patient-Reported Outcome Measurement Information System (PROMIS-10) scores for global physical and mental health; CTT is represented by the Environmental Mastery subscale of the Ryff Psychological Well-Being measure. Although The PROMIS-10 global summary and Environmental Mastery measure do not represent a conception of well-being as generic as Hausman's, they are more generic than the NeuroQol measures. The PROMIS-10 global summary scores limit well-being in terms of physical and mental health, leaving open the population to which it applies. The Environmental Mastery subscale is one of six subscales that make up the Ryff Psychological Well-Being measure; it refers respondents to questions about their feelings of control over their life situation. Like the PROMIS-10, this subscale does not specify a population. These are relatively generic measures.

This article compares applications of these measures at baseline and 17 months later to a population of chronically ill patients and caregivers. The point is to evaluate the measures' susceptibility to response shift according to the restrictiveness of the measures' development. Response shifts effects were inferred using the QOL Appraisal Profile-v2, and they were evaluated using the regression residual modeling approach that I discussed in Chapter 4. The hypothesis animating this study is that the NeuroQol measures are less susceptible to response shift effects than both the PROMIS-10 and the Environmental Mastery measures because they are more restrictive, that is, in Alexandrova's language, more context specific. This study, I suggest, is an approximate test of Alexandrova's proposal. If we conceptualize response shift as indicating heterogeneity, and the NeuroQol unidimensional IRT measures as an instance of contextual well-being, then this study looks to provide insight into whether contextual well-being is more resilient to claims of heterogeneity.

Before discussing the study's findings, it may be helpful to recall the appraisal model's conceptualization of response shift. On this account, response shift must meet three conditions:

1. A discrepancy between what is expected or predicted by the model and what is observed, for example, model misfit or lack of correlation
2. A change in appraisal, that is, recalibration, reprioritization, or reconceptualization

3. Changes in appraisal must be able to explain the unexpected observed change.

It's also necessary to complicate (a bit) my previous explanation of appraisal from Chapter 4. Appraisal can explain unexpected observed change (residual variance) through two pathways: a direct and a moderated route. The moderated route occurs when a change in appraisal is associated with a catalyst (e.g., changes in health, treatment, or life event) and/or a mechanism (e.g., behavioral, cognitive, or affective processes to accommodate changes in catalyst). In this route the change in appraisal mitigates or amplifies the effect of the catalyst. So, for example, the effect of marital status change (a catalyst) on quality of life might be mitigated with an increased appraisal emphasis on independence (Schwartz et al. 2020b). The direct route occurs when a change in appraisal is not associated with a catalyst or a coping mechanism, for example, when quality of life is better than expected due to an increased appraisal emphasis on relationships (Figure 5.1).

The findings from this study support the hypothesis that the unidimensional IRT measures are less sensitive to response shift effects than the multidimensional IRT and CTT measures. At the same time, the study found that unidimensional IRT measures are *not immune* to response shift. Consider: the authors found the suite of NeuroQol instruments did not experience moderated response shift, while the PROMIS-10 and Environmental

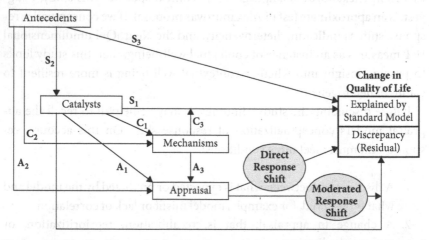

Figure 5.1 The Rapkin and Schwartz theoretical model of direct and moderated response shift.

Mastery measures did. Here is an example of a moderated response shift. The PROMIS-10 global mental health measure showed an association between positive work change (catalyst) and change in relationship focus (appraisal): people who had positive work changes and an increased focus on relationships reported better global mental health. Despite lack of evidence for moderated response shift in the suite of NeuroQol measures, the authors did find evidence of direct response shift, that is, changes in appraisal not associated with catalysts or coping mechanisms. For instance, in the short-form NeuroQoL cognition measures, improved cognitive function was associated with appraisal changes characterized by an increased relationship focus, maintaining roles, and reducing responsibilities. Similarly, for the NeuroQol PAW, improved well-being was associated with appraisal changes characterized by spiritual and relationship focuses, and a decreased emphasis on maintaining roles and reducing responsibilities.

In summary, the contextual measures in this study were resilient against heterogeneity arising from moderated response shift effects. This finding provides some evidence for Alexandrova's proposal that when properly circumscribed, contextual well-being is robust. Nonetheless, these contextual measures were still susceptible to response shift effects through the direct route. In these cases, individuals did come to understand quality of life differently over time, but, interestingly, the changes in appraisal affected the measure similarly across individuals. Schwartz et al. (2020b, 12), write, "The IRT single-domain measures evaluated in this study seemed to change in the same way over time (i.e. in lock-step)." The IRT multidimension measures and the CTT measure were more sensitive to response shift in that different appraisal processes influenced items (questions) differently. What does this mean for Alexandrova's proposal? This study seems to suggest that, even for contextual measures, the construct may change subjective meaning, but these changes may be the same over time for a given population. When the population is unrestricted, we also see change over time, but the impact of these changes is different for different individuals.

What are the implications of this study vis-à-vis Alexandrova's and Hausman's work on well-being? This study is the first of its kind, so whatever inferences we make, we must make them cautiously. Nonetheless, the study provides some evidence that contextual measures of well-being are more robust against instances of heterogeneity than generic measures of well-being. This said, even restrictive unidimensional measures like the NeuroQol instruments are susceptible to changes in the understanding of constructs being measured, and thus response shift effects are relevant to the interpretation of change. Toward the end of the article the authors anticipate those who understand these findings as an incentive to further eliminate changes in appraisal and try to create instruments impervious to response shift. They argue that such efforts are neither feasible nor useful. Reducing changes in appraisal would require detailed instructions to respondents explaining how to constrain their thinking. These instructions would be cumbersome and would reduce, not eliminate, these changes. But importantly, the authors argue that trying to eliminate response shift effects distorts respondents' experiences. This is a counterproductive goal for instruments whose aim is to represent patients' points of view (Schwartz et al. 2020b).

The point that eliminating response shift effects distorts the goal of patient-centered measures is important. It also raises a different set of questions about Alexandrova's proposal. Thus far I've been discussing the measurability of well-being with heterogeneity understood as an obstacle to measurement. This obstacle led Alexandrova to consider a way of limiting heterogeneity while still measuring what we can refer to as "well-being," albeit contextualized to kinds of people in particular situations. But when is limiting heterogeneity effectively distorting well-being? I don't think there is a one-size-fits-all answer to this question. Some measurement purposes will require more contextualized instruments than others, and this reflects current practice. As I have argued elsewhere (McClimans and Browne 2011), determining how much is needed where is inevitably a matter of epistemic and ethical judgment, which means sometimes we will make the wrong judgments. But as I argued in the previous chapter, assuming invariance (or homogeneity) can undermine fitness for purpose. Measuring with instruments that aren't fit for purpose simply to fulfill the goal of measurement—or avoid the possibility of mistakes—is epistemically and ethically problematic.

One of the purposes we should consider is the purpose of patient-centered measures as opposed to other measures of well-being. As I argued in Chapter 2, patient-centered measures are relevantly different from other measures of well-being in their commitment to representing patients' perspectives. And as I argued in Chapter 3, this places them at odds with some of Alexandrova's agenda. This tension emerges again here. Alexandrova contextualizes well-being and generalizes it to a particular kind of people, but patient-centered measures while interested in populations are equally concerned to capture patients' points of view. Patient-centered measures and Alexandrova's proposal for contextual well-being come closest to agreement in unidimensional IRT measures. But what this agreement amounts to changes depending on whether we look at it from the perspective of contextual well-being or patient-centered measures. For contextual well-being the takeaway seems to be the resilience of these instruments. For patient-centered measures, the takeaway seems to be the susceptibility to response shift effects even when measures are developed with restrictive methods. If we take seriously Schwartz and colleagues' (2020b) point that eliminating response shift effects is both not feasible and not useful (and I do), then Alexandrova's proposal seems to sit at one end of a continuum of measures, some more and some less restrictive, but all sensitive to the kind of heterogeneity that response shift and response initiation represent.

5.2. Response Shift Redux

In both of Hausman and Alexandrova's proposals heterogeneity is a characteristic of well-being constructs. That is, when they consider heterogeneity, they are concerned with a version of the question "What is well-being?" This underlying question is reflected in the kinds of considerations they make: Is well-being heterogeneous? Is it all-things-considered or contextualized? Is it flourishing or preferences or subjective well-being? Rapkin and Schwartz (2021) have a more complicated approach to heterogeneity. In their most recent work, they separate patient-centered constructs like quality of life from what they take to be the source of heterogeneity, which Rapkin and Schwartz conceive as response shift. They (2021, 3359) write, "Response shift represents a change in individual perspective—distinct from change in level of QOL but nonetheless meaningful." As Rapkin, Schwartz, and colleagues' work has matured, it's become clearer that they understand quality of life and appraisal as two distinct constructs with two distinct measures. Indeed, they have suggested that measures of quality of life and measures of appraisal represent two distinct types of measurement, psychometric and idiometric, respectively (Schwartz et al. 2020). Nonetheless, their work on appraisal assumes and sometimes makes explicit their belief that "in the appraisal paradigm, QOL can only be understood as encompassing each individuals' unique point of view" (Rapkin and Schwartz 2021, 3359) or as they put it in 2004 (Schwartz and Rapkin 2004, 4), "There is no QOL without an individual's appraisal." In this section, I want to get clearer on the proposal the appraisal approach suggests for the meaning of patient-centered constructs such as quality of life and their relationship to heterogeneity. If changes in patient-centered measures are distinct from changes in individual perspective, in what sense do constructs like quality of life need appraisal?

In Schwartz and Rapkin's (2004; Rapkin and Schwartz 2004) early work on appraisal they were focused on the implications of appraisal on patient-centered measures of quality of life. Thus, they wrote articles like "Reconsidering the Psychometrics of Quality of Life Assessment in Light of Response Shift and Appraisal" (Schwartz and Rapkin 2004). This is a fascinating article that aims to reconceive the psychometric properties of quality of life measures in light of a commitment to legitimating some forms of measurement heterogeneity (or, as they refer to it, "variance"). The article revolves around the idea of a "contingent true score." The contingent true score is Schwartz and Rapkin's answer to the true score, which I discussed briefly in Chapters 1 and 2. But in their article, the idea of a "true score" goes beyond what I discussed earlier to encompass an ideal of measurement, an ideal "fundamental in all psychometric models" (Schwartz and Rapkin 2004, p. 2). Here the true score represents an ideal of invariance, specifically invariance in the meaning of the questions on a patient-centered measure and their relationship to the construct. If these invariances hold, then ceteris paribus observed scores can be considered estimates of true scores across people and time.

Schwartz and Rapkin (2004) argue that the true score ideal is wrong for patient-centered measures. They cash out this claim with a three-way distinction among types of measures: performance, perception, and evaluation-based measures. Schwartz and Rapkin argue that for performance measures (think math tests) and perception measures (think personality tests) the relationship between the questions and the construct remains the same over time and individuals. Accordingly, these measures live up to the true score ideal. The difference, they argue, between performance and perception measures is the role of human judgment. When people answer math test questions, human judgment plays no role in the correct or incorrect answer (in math when people say "round," the convention is to round the final result only). When people answer questions on personality tests, however, human judgment does play a role in terms of, for instance, what behaviors individuals attend to in answering the questions. But, Schwartz and Rapkin (2004) argue, this use of judgment is not intrinsic to the personality constructs. In other words, varying attentiveness doesn't change the meaning of the construct, and to this point, over time, observer ratings should converge. Thus, there are correct and incorrect answers to personality test questions as well as math tests. Even if perception is required to get personality tests off the ground, they argue, it doesn't change the relationship between the questions and the construct.[4]

For Schwartz and Rapkin (2004) evaluative measures (think patient-centered measures) do not live up to the true score ideal. For evaluative constructs such as quality of life, human judgment is "absolutely intrinsic to the phenomenon of interest" (Schwartz and Rapkin 2004, 3). The example they give is quality of life of cancer patients. Cancer patients may interpret the questions on a quality of life measure in any of a number of ways, drawing on different frames of reference, contrasts, and so on. Of these different interpretations, Schwartz and Rapkin (2004, 3) write, "Their answers are no more or less 'true' if they adopt one of these standards over the others. There really is no 'wrong' answer" (Schwartz and Rakin 2004, 3). For evaluative constructs, the relationship between questions and construct is contingent on respondents' appraisal. The ideal of the true score is undermined. Accordingly, we should substitute contingent true scores for true scores when measuring evaluative constructs.

As I discussed above, Schwartz and Rapkin tend to think about a true score as an ideal that represents invariance in the relationship between questions and construct. Similarly, it's useful to think about a contingent true score as an ideal representing variance in the relationship between questions and construct. For Rapkin and Schwartz the source of the variance characteristic of this ideal is not found within the well-being construct, but rather within individual subjective perspectives. Unlike Hausman and Alexandrova, the questions Rapkin, Schwartz, and colleagues are concerned with are not versions of "What is quality of life?" Instead, they are interested in versions of the question "What is response shift?" This question led them to consider appraisal as a possible answer. When Rapkin and Schwartz (2021) consider heterogeneity, they source it within subjective perspectives associated with appraisal.

Schwartz, Rapkin, and colleagues conceptualize appraisal as distinct from patient-centered constructs like quality of life. The distinction between appraisal and quality of life is strengthened and developed over the course of a few papers (Schwartz et al. 2007; Schwartz et al. 2021; Rapkin and Schwartz 2021), but is most forcefully made in their article "Capturing Patient Experience: Does Quality of Life Appraisal Entail a New Class of Measurement?" (Schwartz et al. 2020). In this article they move away from their earlier concern with how appraisal affects the psychometrics of quality of life measures, to concerns about the theoretical and statistical implications of appraisal measures themselves. In making the conceptual case for the distinction between appraisal and quality of life, Schwartz et al. rely on the distinction between psychometric and clinimetric measures on the one hand, and idiometric measures on the other. Psychometric or reflective measurement models, they argue, aim to measure a latent variable by asking questions, the answers of which are taken to "reflect" or be caused by the latent variable. For instance, if depression is being measured using a psychometric model, then the answers to the questions about depression are understood as reflecting levels of depression. Question choice (item selection) for psychometric measures, they argue further, aims for construct unidimensionality and internal consistency. The idea is to choose questions that cover a tightly knit, popular (frequently endorsed) part of the construct to obtain robust results. Patient-centered measures are typically modeled as psychometric measures. The common contrast with psychometric measurement models is clinimetric or formative models. Clinimetric measures identify clinical phenomena (not latent traits). The answers to clinimetric questions are taken to cause changes in the phenomena rather than reflect a construct. Virginia Apgar's (1953) score to evaluate newborn health is an example of a formative measure. The indicators, appearance, pulse, grimace, activity, and respiration, are together taken to provide a profile of a baby's health. Clinimetric measures are not concerned with unidimensionality and internal consistency, as psychometric models are, but, nonetheless, both types of measurement model assume the true score ideal.

Appraisal, as Schwartz et al. (2020) argue, does not fit the psychometric model used in quality of life research; nor does the clinimetric model used for clinical phenomena such as newborn health. Rather, their findings (from empirical studies using appraisal measures) suggest what they call an idiometric measurement model. The authors understand idiometric measures as assessing a construct, but one whose dimensions may be contingent on external variables. The idiometric model thus assumes the contingent true score ideal. To be sure, the authors note, not all cognitive processes are idiosyncratic. Their work with appraisal measures has uncovered correlations of appraisal items across population samples. But they have also found distinct themes in each sample, and the point of their research in this area is that differences in cognitive processes matter—even when the effect size is small.[5] Thus, there are cognitive processes that are sometimes shared across population and time, but also processes that are unique. They argue that a new measurement model is needed to capture and make sense of these differences. Schwartz et al. (2020, 2) write:

> This pattern of findings may suggest that there are shared and unique ways that appraisal items co-vary across patient groups, perhaps due to item content, sample composition or human experience. One has to determine in each assessment context whether and how observations hang together and make sense.

The authors have more to say about the statistical and applied properties of idiometric measures, but for my purposes it is enough to illustrate the distinction they make between psychometric measures of quality of life, on the one hand, and idiometric measures of appraisal, on the other. The former assumes homogeny across people and time, while the latter seeks to identify heterogeny. Another quote drives this point home:

> In contrast to psychometric conceptualizations of measurement structure and construct validity which are posited to be universal properties of the measure itself, we believe that appraisal-measure validation involves the behavior of a measure in-context. These individual cognitive processes are thus posited to be non-ergodic, that is they differ across people and change over time (i.e., non-homogeneous across people and non-stationary over time). (Schwartz et al. 2020, 2)

This proposal places heterogeneity in the subjective perspectives associated with appraisal while leaving patient-centered constructs to the mercies of psychometric measurement. Once patient-centered constructs have been metrologically separated from quality of life appraisal, it can make sense to write, "Response shift represents a change in individual perspective— distinct from change in level of QOL but nonetheless meaningful" (Rapkin and Schwartz 2021, 3359). Yet, as I discussed earlier, Schwartz and Rapkin continue to insist that patient-centered constructs such as quality of life can only be understood in light of appraisal, that is, subjective perspectives. They write, "In the appraisal paradigm, QOL can only be understood as encompassing each individuals' unique point of view" (Rapkin and Schwartz 2021, 3359) or "There is not QOL without an individual's appraisal"

(Schwartz and Rapkin 2004, 2). In both passages they connect our ability to understand or grasp quality of life with appraisal. But if we can only grasp quality of life through appraisal, then how can changes in appraisal be distinct from changes in quality of life?

To my knowledge Schwartz and Rapkin do not address this question. But I suggest we might conceptualize the distinction they make between appraisal and patient-centered constructs along the same lines that we conceptualize a reporting function from a latent trait (Oswald 2008).[6] A reporting function is a cognitive process that translates construct assessments into answers on a questionnaire. Importantly, the reporting function doesn't impact a respondent's assessment of the construct being measured; it just translates that assessment into an answer to a question. Mark Fabian (2022) explains, using an example from Ed Diener and Richard Lucas (1999). Two respondents might assess their life satisfaction identically, but still report it differently on a questionnaire. One respondent might judge life satisfaction as at 8 on a scale from 1 to 10, and the other might judge it at 6 on the same scale. The difference is not the amount of life satisfaction but rather their reporting function, which translates their assessment of life satisfaction into an answer on the questionnaire. In the example, personality traits motivate the different reporting functions. The respondent who gave the answer of 8 is an extrovert, and the person who answered 6 is an introvert.

I am not suggesting here that appraisal can be lumped in with personality traits (see Rapkin et al. 2017). What I am suggesting is that thinking of appraisal along the lines of a reporting function is one way of making sense of two issues (1) there is no quality of life without appraisal and (2) changes in appraisal are distinct from changes in quality of life. If we do think that way, then we can make sense of the idea that we need appraisal to grasp quality of life because it is only through this cognitive process that respondents can translate their assessment of quality of life into an answer about it. On the other hand, quality of life can be understood as distinct from appraisal because two people with the same assessment of their quality of life can respond differently to the same question about it. Perhaps there is another way of making sense of this distinction, but this is the strongest and clearest interpretation I can currently give it.

Nonetheless, I am skeptical of the coherence of this interpretation. The interpretative strategy above trades on two different understandings of patience-centered constructs like quality of life. First, there is quality of life qua construct or latent trait (what respondents assess internally), and second there is quality of life qua appraisal (the answers respondents give to questions about quality of life). The first understanding is the version of quality of life that we might say resides within respondents. This is the quality of life upon which respondents make an initial assessment. The second understanding of quality of life is the version that "lives" outside respondents as answers to questions. This is respondents' assessment of quality of life translated onto a scale. On this interpretation, there is a construct or latent trait and two respondent assessments of this construct. One assessment is internal and private; the other is external and public. Appraisal is part of the external, public reporting function of quality of life. This is how we can say there is no quality of life without appraisal. But what about when we say changes in quality of life are different from changes in appraisal? If "changes in appraisal" refers to changes in the public reporting function of quality of life, what does "changes in quality of life" refer to? Does it refer to the internal, private assessment of the construct or latent trait? Or does it refer to the construct or latent trait itself, that is, the construct prior to respondent assessment of it?

Both options seem problematic. If "changes in quality of life" refers to the internal, private assessment of quality of life, it's not clear how we get access to this assessment without also turning it into an appraisal of quality of life. That is, once we ask respondents questions about their assessment of quality of life, we will also activate appraisal processes.[7] Alternatively, if "changes in quality of life" refers to the construct prior to respondent assessment, it's equally unclear how we gain access to it. On the one hand, as I discussed in Chapter 1, we lack "gold standards" or external criteria of patient-centered constructs (Hunt 1997). On the other hand, when we ask caregivers or clinicians about quality of life of their dependents or patients, they regularly underestimate it (they bring into play their own appraisal processes) (Crocker et al. 2015). Indeed, as Rapkin and Schwartz discuss (2019), health researchers aren't explicit about defining where the "expected" values of patient-centered constructs come from. Often they seem to be made on assumptions about the relationship between health and quality of life, but response shift research was developed in part to illustrate the complexity of these assumptions.

When Schwartz and Rapkin make a distinction between changes in appraisal and changes in quality of life, they suggest that quality of life is something that we can measure and understand independent of the cognitive processes we use to talk about it. These cognitive processes, such as invoking standards of comparisons, experience sampling, and frames of reference, are ways that our values and assumptions about patient-centered constructs are applied to them. For instance, when I understand a question about my limitations pursuing leisure activities in terms of reading rather than gardening, I am expressing a value; when I compare my health to others my age rather than my own health last year, I'm assuming a comparator that is important and meaningful to me. This raises an epistemic problem. Is it possible to measure or understand patient-centered constructs independent of our values and assumptions about them? In Chapter 1 I argued that it is not. I argued that although philosophers of science, hermeneuticists, and health researchers have tried to separate values and assumptions from science, this strategy is not a promising one. In fact, I argued that values and assumptions are conditions for the possibility of knowledge; we cannot peel back the values and assumptions implicit in quality of life to get at a value-free (appraisal-free) version of it. Yet this is what (at least on my interpretation) Rapkin and Schwartz seem to require if changes in quality of life are distinct from changes in appraisal.

Finally, I want to raise a possible ethical problem with the distinction Schwartz and Rapkin make between changes in quality of life and changes in appraisal. As I discussed in Chapter 4, Schwartz and Rapkin have consistently argued that response shift effects should not be conceptualized as bias; rather these effects are meaningful information. Indeed, in some contexts response shift effects are the point of therapy, a feature not a bug. Yet if changes in quality of life are distinct from changes in appraisal (response shift effects) in terms of their measurement models and (the philosopher in me wants to say) their ontology, then it's easy to see why response shift would be conceptualized as bias. The FDA (FDA 2009, 2023), the United Kingdom (NHS 2023), Denmark (Egholm et al. 2023), and the Organization for Economic Co-operation and Development (2017) are interested in patient-centered constructs, *not* response shift. If it's possible to isolate these constructs against the complications of response shift effects, then all the better—except, of course, that in doing so we take away the "patient-centered" part of these constructs. For if we remove subjective perspectives (appraisal) from measuring these constructs, then we lose what is ethically unique. I think separating appraisal from patient-centered constructs is ethically and epistemically problematic.

In Hausman and Alexandrova's work what matters is well-being as an object of science. Both consider well-being and worry about heterogeneity and its implications for measuring well-being. For Hausman heterogeneity makes measurement largely unusable for health policy; for Alexandrova heterogeneity can be tamed if we circumscribe our measures to specific people in particular situations. For both, heterogeneity is construed as an obstacle. In the work of Schwartz, Rapkin, and colleagues, heterogeneity is found in subjective perspectives, or as they refer to it, appraisal. In their work heterogeneity is also an obstacle, but it is an obstacle that is overcome with more measurement. Subjective perspectives are isolated from patient-centered constructs and then measured in their own right. While both subjective perspectives and patient-centered constructs are measurable, they take on different measurement models: patient-centered constructs are psychometric or reflexive, while perspectives are idiometric. In the next section I argue that heterogeneity is not an obstacle to measuring patient-centered constructs; rather, heterogeneity makes patient-centered measurement possible. Making this argument will take us once again on a journey into Gadamer's hermeneutics.

5.3. Hermeneutics Redux

In this section I flesh out a hermeneutic response to the question I've been considering throughout this chapter, that is, the conceptualization of patient-centered constructs and their relationship to heterogeneity. Nonetheless, I'll illustrate that on my hermeneutic account the relationship in question is not one between patient-centered constructs and heterogeneity, but rather between patient-centered constructs and the testimony and responses of people with disabilities, patients, and other ill people. On my account, heterogeneity falls out of the relationship; heterogeneity is an inescapable feature of studying patient-centered constructs such as quality of life. To understand why this is so, we need to dig a bit into Gadamer's ontological vision because differences in understanding, say, quality of life aren't for him simply a matter of differing subjective perspectives, but can disclose what quality of life is. In fact, on Gadamer's account understanding has nothing to do with subjectivity. His vision thus challenges attempts like Rapkin and Schwartz's to separate well-being constructs from subjective perspectives on them. For instance, when I come to understand that quality of life is not synonymous with health, when I come to understand that a good-quality life includes diverse bodies with diverse abilities, then I also come to know what quality of life is—not what I want or wish it to be, but what it really and truly is.

Gadamer, after all, was a realist (Wachterhauser 2002). It's now time to explore this claim further.

Our exploration may benefit from briefly acknowledging the historical position Gadamer occupies vis-à-vis a philosophical discussion of "ontology," or what we might think of as the science of reality. Gadamer takes to heart George Wilhelm Friedrich Hegel's (1809/1979) criticism of Immanuel Kant's (1781/1999) distinction between the "noumenal," that is, the world as it is in itself, and "phenomenal," that is, the world as we observe it. Gadamer thus agrees with Hegel that the noumenal realm is nonsensical: either the noumenal realm is beyond reason, in which case we can't know it or discuss it, or it is within reason, and then it isn't distinguishable from the phenomenal realm. The upshot of this agreement is that Gadamer rejects the idea of a reality that lies beyond human interests and concerns; the real world *is* the world in which we live and work. Moreover and importantly, for Gadamer (and Heidegger) it is through our interests and concerns that reality and our own selves are disclosed to us. The nature of this disclosure, for Gadamer, is understanding. Here are a few examples.

I love horses. Although I rode intermittently as a child and young adult, I am only recently in the position to dedicate myself to this interest. Like any serious hobby, horse riding and horse ownership are a world unto itself. Over the last few years, this interest led me down paths of engagement with horses, barns, trainers, and shows. As I come to understand the horse world, I also come to understand more about myself. For instance, jumping a horse often seems to require bravery or brash self-confidence. I often lack both. I enjoy dressage, which reminds me of philosophy—the precision, the detail—and this in turn has made me think that I am more of a philosopher than I once thought. The relationship between horse owners and barn managers is one fraught with potential conflict (turn-out, feeding, ring use, etc.). I hate conflict, so this relationship is a constant, if often latent, stress.

What does this example illustrate? Clearly, it shows how my interest in horses revealed a reality with which I was previously unfamiliar, and in doing so it revealed more about who I am. But one might object that the horse world existed before I got interested in it! How does this example help motivate the point that reality is disclosed though our interests and concerns? Remember that for Gadamer understanding is dialogic, so when I say I came to understand my way around the horse world, what I mean is that I entered into a dialogue with the horse world, a dialogue that is characterized by unstandardized questions. I discussed these kinds of questions in Chapter 4. To be sure, horses and lessons and shows and barns and horse people existed before I became interested in them, but the Gadamerian point here is that this world doesn't exist without language, without the give-and-take, back-and-forth of unstandardized questions and answers. So, yes, the horse world existed before my interest in it, but it doesn't exist independent of *human* interest. When I entered this dialogue I became a part of it—both the dialogue and the horse world. As a part of this dialogue I learned about the horse world, but I also contributed to what it is. We saw an example of this contribution in the previous chapter. When I asked, "What should I do when Toni won't listen in lessons?" I learned that "doing" doesn't start when I get into the saddle, and improving my riding skills isn't the only answer to my question. But equally, what I should do in the saddle remained important to me, and thus I contributed in a small way to what this world is, that is, a world with a rider like me who has this question. Similarly, when I think about jumping horses, what I have learned so far is that it takes either bravery or brash self-confidence, virtues I some-times lack. Yet I keep wondering if there is not another way to understand jumping, a way that might better comport with who I am. Might repetition overcome bravery? So I keep jumping small jumps. Over and over. To this end, I am not simply a sponge in the horse world, but also a contributor, however small and local, to what this world *is*.

What I am saying can be summarized by Gadamer (2013, 468 and 490) when he writes, "Being that can be understood is language." Much has been written on what precisely Gadamer might mean by this claim (e.g., Lammi 1991; Wachterhauser 1994, 1999; Rorty 2004; Lynch 2021), and it is beyond the scope of this book to resolve *that* debate. Instead, I'd like to dis-cuss what it doesn't mean, about which there is more consensus, and then sketch out what I take to be a reasonable interpretation. First, Gadamer's claim doesn't mean that language determines reality. I can't say something and bibbidy-bobbidy-boo make it so. I can still be wrong about what I say; we can be wrong about what we believe. This is a familiar point in the his-tory of science. We once had a geocentric model of the solar system. We were wrong. If I say, "It doesn't matter what we wear in the county horse show be-cause it's local and just for fun," that doesn't mean if we rock up to the show with a dirty pony, training jodhpurs, and a T-shirt all will be fine. It really does matter what you wear, local and for fun notwithstanding. But being wrong doesn't entail, on Gadamer's view, that there is a "reality" that stands behind language and dictates its terms. Rather, being wrong on Gadamer's view indicates a place where different, relevant parts of our language—our thoughts, meanings, and representations—fail to cohere.

Second, "Being that can be understood is language" doesn't mean that language paints a canvas on an unintelligible reality. Remember, this is not a Kantian picture of noumenal reality as the world is in itself on one side and phenomenal reality as we experience it on the other. Instead, as Greg Lynch argues, Gadamer's picture is one where there is an isomorphism between language and the world language describes. Lynch (2021, 1003) puts the point like this: "There can be no necessary gap between the way language presents reality to us and the way reality is." Language thus discloses an intelligible world to us; language doesn't make the world intelligible. At the same time, language can enhance the world's intelligibility. Language can describe the world in a such a way as to make it more meaningful to us, but language can also get it wrong. When Sontag (1978) described the world as consisting of the kingdom of the well and the kingdom of the sick, she enhanced the world's intelligibility; when we conceptualized the solar system as geocentric, we confused it. To reiterate, when Lynch says there is no gap between language and reality, he doesn't mean everything we say is true. What he means is there is no aspect of reality impervious to language. People with disabilities, patients, and other ill people can enhance the intelligibility of patient-centered constructs, but they can also confuse them. This is why qualitative research needs epistemic dialogue and why changes in appraisal need criteria such as those offered by recalibration, reprioritization, and reconceptualization.

The relationship Gadamer envisions between language and the world—the relationship I envision between the testimony and responses of people with disabilities, patients, and other ill people and patient-centered constructs—is characterized by both autonomy and dependence. The world is separate from language, and yet it is dependent on language to make it meaningful. If we apply this thought to patient-centered constructs, we can say they are independent of what we might say about them, and yet we need testimony, expertise, and respondent answers to make them meaningful. Think about patient-centered constructs or latent traits. They are not identical with respondents' appraisals of them, but as I argued in the previous section, we need appraisals to make them meaningful. To motivate this vision, I find Gadamer's discussion of art helpful. Consider a play. Plays are brought to life when they are performed; it is only through their performance that a play takes on a concrete existence. For Gadamer the audience is essential to a work of art. Without an audience works of art cannot be interpreted, and thus they don't have a meaningful existence for us. If an audience is an essential condition of a work of art, then an audience is necessary not only for the performing arts but also for the non-performing arts. Just as music must be heard, paintings must be viewed. Art is brought to life through an audience; it is thus dependent on an audience. But art also exerts normative authority over its audience. It is thus also independent of its audience. Similarly, patient-centered constructs are made meaningful through respondents' appraisals of them; they are thus dependent on respondents. But as I discussed in Chapter 3, not just any respondent interpretation will do. We can question these interpretations and discuss what interpretation is best; thus these constructs are also independent from us.

According to Gadamer, art's independence is derived through its representational capacity. Here Gadamer argues that art imitates reality. This reality is then presented to an audience as a claim to truth. Gadamer's account, however, does not suggest that works of art accurately depict aspects of reality. Rather, works of art reveal to an audience a possible truth about reality, a truth that is overlooked, forgotten, or difficult to unearth in everyday life. As Alasdair MacIntyre (1981) writes, portrait painters from the 14th to the 17th century learned to reveal with their art the virtues that lay behind the faces of their sitting subjects. This disclosure was partially accomplished by Rembrandt through the technique of impasto, which layered paint in such a way as to stand out from the canvas. These raised surfaces allowed Rembrandt to play with reflected light and textures to create realistic likenesses. Other artists accomplish revelations through appropriation, exaggeration, abstraction, and so on. In its capacity to make a claim to truth, art imparts knowledge to its audience and challenges the audience to respond to these revelations. But—crucially—the content of this normative authority is not independent of the specific audience who watches, views, or listens to it. Recall that for Gadamer an audience is essential to the meaningful existence of a work of art. This means that the audience contributes to the content of the truth claim that art makes through their interpretation of it. This interpretation in turn depends on the relevance that the art has to a particular audience. This relationship between art and its audience is similar to the relationship respondents and health researchers have to patient-centered constructs through epistemic dialogue.

In Lynch's (2021) account of Gadamer's realism, he argues that the relationship Gadamer envisions between an audience and art—the relationship I've characterized as autonomy and dependence—is analogous to the relationship Gadamer envisions between language and being. Just as a performance makes a musical score meaningful to us, that is, gives the music a concrete existence, language makes the world meaningful to us, gives it a concrete existence. And just as different performances of the same score performed before different audiences can be differently meaningful, so too can different articulations of the world be differently meaningful. Moreover, the meaning language makes of the world is a claim about truth. It's a claim about how the world is—not simply how I see the world, not simply a subjective perspective. Lynch (2021) helpfully explains Gadamer's truth claim in terms of "factualness" rather than objectivity. For Gadamer things are independent of whether we believe them to be this way or not; thus our interpretation of the world can be better or worse. For instance, we can see the world more clearly, and we can better capture the meaning of a painting. Language and the world are factual, but they are not objective. This means that while there is a way the world is, the way it is isn't independent of human interests. It's only through the application of language oriented toward human interests and concerns that the world takes on a concrete, meaningful existence.

If we apply this claim to patient-centered measurement, then it's possible to talk abstractly about "constructs" and "subjective perspectives" just as we talk abstractly about "language" and the "world" or "performances" and "musical scores," but it's only through application of perspective to construct that we have something we can meaningfully study, investigate, probe, *measure*. The nature of this application is, for Gadamer, dialogic. I discussed Gadamer's dialogic mode of understanding in Chapter 3 to motivate my account of epistemic dialogue during the development of patient-centered constructs. But as I discussed in Chapter 4, patient-centered constructs have a life that continues beyond the development of a measure, a life that continues into the application of these measures on populations through ongoing coordination. I now suggest that this application phase where measures are applied to different populations of respondents has a dialogic function.

Dialogues are for Gadamer characterized by questions and answers. Indeed, on Gadamer's account statements receive their meaning when we understand them as answers to questions. For instance, the sentence "I just bought a pony" takes on a different meaning when understood as the answer to "Do your children ride?" than when understood as the answer to "Where does all your money go?" This doesn't mean, of course, that all statements have preordained questions that dictate their meaning, but rather that if we want to understand a statement, then we must explicitly or implicitly understand it as the answer to some question or another. To be sure, we can misunderstand a statement if we imagine it as the answer to the wrong question. If I say, "I bought a pony!" and you say, "Is this why you never have any money?" and I look at you quizzically, you may (be embarrassed to) realize you understood me incorrectly. I wasn't referring to money when I told you about the new pony, I was talking about a new opportunity for my children. Dialogues are in the business of asking and answering questions about something—about raising children, about what makes for a good quality of life, the meaning of a text. It is through questioning that we come to understand these things. Good interpretations are coherent and respect the truth claim of what we aim to understand.

Schwartz and Rapkin echo Gadamer's sentiment regarding the meaningfulness of answers in light of questions when they argue for the importance of a "backstory." As I quoted them in Chapter 4, "There are many ways to arrive at a rating, but QOL ratings in and of themselves convey no 'backstory' about the process of appraisal. Without this information, it is impossible to understand what a score means or how to validate it" (2004, 4). Schwartz and Rapkin argue that it isn't enough to get answers from respondents. If we want to understand what those answers mean, we need to understand the backstory, or the questions respondents take themselves to be answering. It is understanding respondent answers as the answer to a particular question that gives it meaning. Gadamer adds to their argument the ontological consequences of understanding. The questions and answers that constitute patient-centered measures are oriented toward understanding the construct of interest. While it's true that respondent answers should be understood in light of their questions, it's also true on my account that respondent answers affect what the construct *is*. Indeed, their answers divulge the construct as meaningful. The upshot of the connection Gadamer draws between language and being is that patient-centered constructs *cannot* be measured or studied independent of respondent perspectives or vice versa. Subjective perspectives of people with disabilities, patients, and other ill people impact what these constructs are, and thus perspectives and constructs are connected to one another just as performances and art, language, and world are linked.

In Chapter 1 I suggested that pluralism is built into Gadamer's account of understanding, similar to the role pluralism plays in Chang's coherentism. Gadamer's hermeneutics allows us to learn different though equally legitimate lessons from the same topic of interest. Differences in historical or cultural standpoints as well as practical and theoretical commitments can lead to different but nonetheless valid interpretations. A good quality of life might be living independently even if that means a shorter life; a good quality of life might equally be one that is dependent on extended family. I now want to suggest that this pluralism should be understood similarly to the heterogeneity or variance that philosophers and health researchers discuss vis-à-vis well-being constructs. Alexandrova, Hausman, and Rapkin and Schwartz will agree that a good quality of life means different things to different people and may mean different things over time to the same people. For Gadamer these differences enrich what these constructs are. But the source of these differences (their heterogeneity) doesn't reside in the construct as Hausman and Alexandrova conceptualize it nor does it reside in subjective perspectives as Rapkin, Schwartz, and colleagues conceptualize it. Instead, this pluralism or "heterogeneity" resides in the "in-between" of perspectives and constructs. And for Gadamer it is this in-between, or, we might say, in this application of perspectives to constructs, that constructs, art—the *world*—come into existence for us.

5.4. Conclusion

Philosophers of well-being and health researchers worry about measurability. Heterogeneity is often understood as an obstacle to measurability, as we saw in my discussion of Hausman and Alexandrova. Schwartz, Rapkin, and colleagues' position is more complicated, but in their most recent work patient-centered constructs like quality of life are preserved for nomothetic measurement, and this is done by removing the source of heterogeneity and treating it separately. A hermeneutic account of measurement resists concerns of measurability because it doesn't suppose the answer lies in identifying relatively homogeneous, psychometric, true-score-applicable constructs of well-being. But neither does it think understanding or grasping quality of life is a matter of unearthing subjective perspectives. Rather a hermeneutic account of measurement begins with the bedrock assumption that constructs are subject to pluralism; that is, they are heterogeneous. If we want to measure them, then we can't sidestep, circumscribe, or siphon off heterogeny. Instead we must face it.

The heterogeny present in patient-centered constructs is born from a relationship of autonomy and dependence between constructs and subjective perspectives, between questions and answers. Patient-centered measures have the dual role of both locating respondents within the space of a construct or latent trait *and* facilitating heterogeneity of these same constructs or latent traits. We cannot measure patient-centered constructs without also facilitating heterogeneity; we cannot parcel heterogeneity off. This heterogeneity, this pluralism, is in fact the justification for my conclusion in the previous chapter: patient-centered measures require ongoing coordination.

Coordinating patient-centered measures is never one and done. The very nature of posing questions to respondents necessitates appraisal, and appraisal exposes constructs to time and context sensitivity. Appraisal measures, or something like them, are thus crucial to a hermeneutic account of patient-centered measures. Appraisal measures used in tandem with patient-centered measures can provide an estimate of respondents' understanding of patient-centered constructs. Appraisal brings meaning to respondent answers on patient-centered measures. In other words, appraisal helps us to understand what patient-centered constructs *are*. But, as I discussed at the end of the previous chapter, this doesn't mean every application of patient-centered measures requires redevelopment—this would be impractical. Instead, I envisage appraisal metrics used alongside patient-centered outcomes similar to the way uncertainty budgets are used with primary standards. It's only when we think we can create better patient-centered measures, that is, measures that more aptly reflect the construct without loss of, for instance, responsiveness, usefulness, that we redevelop them.

Some might respond to my argument in this chapter with the suggestion that we stop measuring patient-centered constructs. But why should we stop? There are many reasons why we should *not* stop. Here are just a few. There are practical reasons: they are integrated into many national healthcare systems, for example, in Denmark (Lindström et al. 2023) and the United Kingdom (NHS 2023). Moreover, they've become integral to many applications to the FDA. There are ethical reasons: they provide an opportunity for patient points of view to impact macro-, meso- and micro-level healthcare decision-making. There are epistemic reasons: they increase our knowledge about what constructs such as quality of life and physical functioning *are*.

Patient-centered measures have the capacity to be useful, good, and informative. But it is true that measuring patient-centered constructs is not easy. Certainly, it is not as easy as we hoped it might be. Measuring these constructs facilitates heterogeneity, and heterogeneity has long been thought the enemy of measurement, at least in the well-being sciences. But I think it is important to remember that measurement is rarely easy. Behind the scenes, measuring temperature and time is difficult and complex. And while heterogeneity has been seen as an obstacle to measuring well-being, when we reframe patient-centered measures as needing epistemic dialogue and ongoing coordination, then heterogeneity is less an obstacle than a fact about measurement, one that is continuous with other types of measures, for instance, the measure of time.

This book has argued that facing pluralism or heterogeneity is not only possible, but also practical. The seeds of the practices that make facing it possible are already part of patient-centered measurement. We don't need to reinvent the wheel. Facing heterogeneity is a matter of management, using practices we already have. On the development end of measurement, I've argued we should manage pluralism or heterogeny through epistemic dialogue; on the applied end of measurement, we should manage it through something like appraisal adjuncts and ongoing coordination. Both suggestions come from practices already in use in the field or alterations of such practices. The FDA emphasizes qualitative research, and Denmark's Program PRO (Lindström et al. 2023) included extensive consultation between patient groups and health researchers. To these initiatives, I have added epistemic dialogue. Schwartz, Rapkin, and colleagues have emphasized appraisal adjuncts, and although I agree with their importance and believe they should be used in conjunction with patient-centered measures, I disagree that they should be construed as separate constructs characterized by distinct measurement models. I find more agreement with their arguments about the evaluative nature of patient-centered constructs and the implication that human judgment is intrinsic to these constructs.

In the next chapter of this book I turn to the use of patient-centered measures in medical and pharmaceutical industries. Thus far I've been arguing for an account of patient-centered measures that makes sense of their claim of "representing patient perspectives." I've argued for a hermeneutic account of these measures that gives people with disabilities, patients, and other ill people a substantive role in developing these measures, not simply responding to them. My hope for this account—and what I take to be the aspiration for these instruments—is that it will make the decisions for which these measurement outcomes serve as evidence more sensitive to human needs and interests. But the use of these measures in these industries is a challenge to this hope. As I discussed in Chapter 3, philosophers have recently discussed how medical and pharmaceutical industries can co-opt and exploit efforts to incorporate patient perspectives in drug development (Bueter and Jukola 2020; Holman and Geislar 2018). The concern is that they use the FDA's interest in patient perspectives to bias the discussion at these meetings, and further their own economic interests. Does patient-centered measurement play into the hands of attempts to exploit patient-focused initiatives? I will argue that while patient-focused initiatives, including patient-centered measurement, open opportunities for exploitation, this is not a sufficient reason to give up on them.

6

Industry and Patient-Focused Initiatives

Throughout this book I've championed the attempt to make measures patient-centered. I've argued not only that these instruments can live up to their claim to "represent patient perspectives" but also that they should. Patient-centered measures that ask people with disabilities, patients, and other ill persons about their quality of life, functioning, or other related experiences should recognize the expertise they bring to these questions. On my account this means taking their answers seriously as a claim to truth, a claim about how the world is. Yet philosophical critiques of both patient-centered approaches and hermeneutic inquiry have argued equally that such an approach may be naive.

As I discussed in Chapter 3, contemporary philosophers have noted how pharmaceutical industries can manipulate attempts to make the FDA's regulatory review process more patient centered. Recall that from 2012 to 2015 the FDA, as part of its Patient Focused Drug Development Program, held 24 disease-specific public meetings. These meetings were held to better understand patient perspectives on the clinical significance of drugs under FDA review. Yet, as I noted in Chapter 3, Holman and Geislar argue that at the FDA's meeting to obtain patient perspectives on flibanserin (a drug that was under review to treat female sexual disfunction, or FSD), industry upended the FDA's intentions, and in fact captured the meeting by injecting industry-sponsored patient representatives. In their research, Holman and Geislar found over half the participants at this meeting were associated with the pharmaceutical company that stood to financially benefit from the drug's approval, and nearly three-quarters of the speaking time at the meeting was taken up with these industry-sponsored patient perspectives. Perhaps not surprisingly, the participants associated with the drug company voiced support for the drug's approval. The FDA, which ignored patient affiliations, treated all viewpoints with equal weight. We might say the FDA treated all patient perspectives as representing a claim to truth, as I have suggested we should do. Yet in doing so, Holman and Geisler argue, it was easy for the sponsored participant voices to overshadow non-industry-sponsored ones.

Patient-Centered Measurement. Leah M. McClimans, Oxford University Press. © Oxford University Press 2024.
DOI: 10.1093/oso/9780197572078.003.0007

The latter unanimously resisted thinking about FSD in terms of a biological problem with a pharmaceutical solution. Nonetheless, the FDA summarized the meeting as voicing a general willingness to undertake the risk of medication in order to obtain relief from FSD.

This example illustrates how industry-sponsored participants affected the summary of this public meeting. It also raises questions about the wisdom of using these kinds of public forums and similar efforts to collect patient perspectives to inform policy, clinical significance, or other information. It serves to remind us that relations of power such as those between pharmaceutical industries and sponsored patient representatives can "distort expressions of needs and misdirect goals and aspirations" (Warnke 2014, 648). The questions this example raises about patient-focused initiatives are illustrative of the criticisms philosophers such as Habermas (1977) and feminist theorists (e.g., Code 2003) have long levied against Gadamerian hermeneutics. Their worry, similar to Holman and Geisler's worry, is that individual expressions of perspective may be given in the service of self-interest (through coercion), self-aggrandizement, and institutional ideology rather than the pursuit of truth. Moreover, when we treat such expressions on par with others as possibly true, we risk perpetuating and codifying those interests.

Nonetheless, although aware of these concerns, Gadamer is unwavering in his commitment to taking claims seriously as claims to truth (Wellmer 1974). Understanding, on Gadamer's account, places epistemic and ethical demands on us, not psychological or historical ones; thus we shouldn't explain away participants' claims. Epistemically, when we orient ourselves toward understanding, we aim to understand *what* something is, not why people say what they say. Understanding is not a matter of going behind language to understand its psychological or historical roots. Ethically, for Gadamer the alternative to this relationship of possible truth is to objectify or psychologize those with whom we converse. Consider objectification. In the flibanserin meeting, the FDA could have objectified the industry-sponsored participants. In doing so it could have discounted or devalued their perspectives by reasoning that their perspectives were a symptom or effect of an underlying cause, for instance, receiving money for participation (Warnke 2014; see also Holman and Bruner 2015). Alternatively, we can psychologize our interlocuters. We can discount their contribution by claiming to know better what they really mean. In her discussion of Fricker's interpretation of *The Talented Mr. Ripley*, Warnke (2014) gives the example of Herbert Greenleaf's behavior toward Marge Sherwood. When Sherwood brings her suspicions about Ripley to Greenleaf, he dismisses them as the fluff and nonsense of female intuition and reconceives them as an expression of disappointment over how little Marge really knew Dickie.

Objectifying or psychologizing our interlocuters is problematic for Gadamer. In both cases we abdicate our relationship with them; as Warnke (2014) so aptly puts it: we pull rank. We refuse to treat our interlocuters as equals. When we pull rank, *we* determine the significance of our interlocuters' contributions—you're only saying this because you were sponsored by industry. Or your outburst is misplaced—what you really mean is you wish you knew my son better. When we pull rank, we effectively decide from what and whom we can learn. So: we can't learn from industry-sponsored participants or women, but we can learn from unsponsored participants and men? We don't need to go deep into hermeneutic theory to see the problem with this approach: we often make mistakes about where learning can take place. Gadamer's hermeneutics, however, helps diagnose why we make these mistakes. When we pull rank, we think we protect ourselves from perpetuating and codifying interests that undermine truth, but we also protect ourselves from examining our own prejudice and bias.

Keeping comfortable in the name of protecting oneself from ignorance and immorality is a familiar power play. Perhaps it is not always unjustified, but it risks the shadow of ultracrepidarianism. As I said at the beginning of Chapter 1, this book is a story about how to avoid that kind of hubris; in this chapter I'm going to continue to argue that patient-centered measures are not only possible, but epistemically important and morally virtuous. This position, however, does not suppose the threat pharmaceutical industries pose isn't real. It is real. But the position I develop characterizes this threat in terms of their influence over the questions we ask about medical products. I argue the best way to resist this influence is to double down on epistemic dialogue. To make this argument I provide examples of the pharmaceutical industry's influence, first, by illustrating how measure development can be used to further their goals, then, by looking at how industries wield influence beyond measurement to the production, evaluation, and dissemination of medical information. I argue that their influence, whether over measurement, clinical trials, scientific publications, or regulation, has the effect of obscuring questions of values (harms and benefits) and economics (profits and losses) while highlighting a narrow version of scientific rigor. This interest in a particular representation of scientific rigor benefits these industries. So what should we do? I end this chapter considering the relative merits of pulling rank over doubling down on dialogue. I argue epistemic dialogue wins. I hope you will agree.

6.1. Industry and Measure Development: Two Examples

The example Holman and Geisler (2018) offer from the FDA's flibanserin meeting provides an illustration of the possible danger pharmaceutical industries pose in determining clinical significance. I use this example in Chapter 3 to complicate the picture of qualitative research during the development of patient-centered measures. I argue there that qualitative research allows us to foreground the perspectives of people with disabilities, patients, and other ill people when developing patient-centered measures. This contribution from qualitative research is important and valuable. Yet epistemically and ethically responsible measures cannot simply acquiesce to these perspectives; rather I argue health researchers need to understand these perspectives and that only happens when they ask questions about them. In asking questions and listening to answers—by participating in epistemic dialogue—between researchers and those with firsthand experience, we move toward a better understanding about quality of life with epilepsy or prostate cancer or whatever is being investigated. In the examples that follow, epistemic dialogue from diverse points of view becomes only more important in the attempt to limit the kind of capture Holman and Geisler describe.

In this section, I provide two examples of pharmaceutical industry's potential influence on measurement. These examples together form a picture of how decisions made during measure development—decisions often labeled "scientific" or "patient centered"—can be used in ways that may in fact undermine science and patients' interests. These examples broadly involve increasing the sensitivity or changing the range of patient-centered measures. Before digging into the details of these examples, a short introduction to measurement sensitivity and range might be helpful.

It is important to understand that just as seeking public input into topics about which people have expertise is part of good social and medical science, so is it part of good science to ensure that a measure has an appropriate sensitivity and range. Indeed, the natural sciences require measuring instruments to be sufficiently sensitive to the range of the quantity under investigation; health science is no different. Yet, as I will illustrate, questions of sensitivity and range can be part of a decision process that benefits pharmaceutical industries and those researchers whose work depends on their contracts.

To get a sense of the complications, consider sensitivity. Sensitivity is the smallest absolute amount of change that can be detected by an instrument. When we want to measure small changes in temperature, for instance, we need more sensitive thermometers than we do when we want to measure larger changes in temperature. Why? Because smaller changes in temperature won't register on less sensitive measures. Similarly, if we want to measure fine-grained changes in quality of life, we need a more sensitive measure than when our measurement goals are less discriminating. Nonetheless, measurement sensitivity can be manipulated to, for instance, illustrate a treatment benefit that is of questionable social value or inflate the numbers of diagnoses. As Justin Biddle (2016) notes, one of the causes of overdiagnosis is the increased sensitivity of diagnostic tests. These tests diagnose disease that will rarely if ever progress to symptoms or early disease, but they do justify expensive treatments.

Now consider range. The range of a thermometer refers to the difference between the minimum and maximum temperatures the instrument can read. A common range for a household thermometer is −10 to 110 Celsius, but the average range of a clinical thermometer is 35 to 42 Celsius. These differences in range correspond to the purposes to which these instruments are put. Similarly, patient-centered measures can cover different ranges of a construct for different measurement purposes. Some measures cover general quality of life; these measures have a wide range. Other measures are more specific, targeting, for example, the higher-functioning ranges of quality of life. Tailoring a measure's range to the measurement context is good science, but it can also be manipulated. Outcomes from instruments with a range that targets high functioning can be used as evidence for healthcare needs. Yet these healthcare needs may only be relevant when we limit our investigation to a high-functioning population. When we look at the overall spectrum of functioning, the needs of high-functioning adults may pale in importance. It's as if we only looked at the education needs of upper-middle-class children. We might find that some are worse off because they don't have access to private education. But the relevance of this factor for the overall population requires us to look at the educational needs of a larger spectrum of the economy (see, e.g., Daniels 1981). If measures with limited ranges seduce us into absolute thinking, they can lead to the proliferation of disease categories, overtreatment, and the unwise use of resources.

6.1.1. Sensitivity and Responsiveness

When we talk about patient-centered measures, questions of sensitivity are bound up with questions of responsiveness and interpretability. Responsiveness refers to an instrument's sensitivity to change. It is one of the core psychometric properties of patient-centered measures. Responsiveness is defined as change over time; the COSMIN checklist defines it as "longitudinal validity" (Mokkink et al. 2019). Interpretability, on the other hand, refers to clinically meaningful change (Guyatt 2000). There are different methods of determining interpretability, for instance, distribution-based methods and anchor-based methods, as well as combinations of the two (e.g., Jaeschke et al. 1989; Cella et al. 2002; for a critique of anchor-based methods see McClimans 2011). But regardless of the method, for many health researchers clinically meaningful change in the context of patient-centered measures must refer to change that is meaningful to people with disabilities, patients, and other ill persons. This is why public meetings such as those held by the FDA are important to measurement design and not simply an issue for drug development and approval. These meetings provide qualitative evidence of clinical changes that are important. When we develop patient-centered measures, what we want are measures that are meaningfully sensitive to changes in the construct being measured. Thus, to justify the need for a more sensitive measure, we need to show that its sensitivity undergirds clinically meaningful change.

Although there are complex methodological techniques for achieving interpretability and measuring responsiveness (e.g., Mokkink et al. 2019), the concept of sensitivity in patient-centered measures is quite simple: it comes down to the number and kinds of questions posed to respondents. For example, single-question scales—scales that ask only one question—are limited in sensitivity since they must divide rich constructs, like spasticity, into only a few levels (Hobart et al. 2007). Multi-question scales are more sensitive because rich constructs are broken down into a greater number of components. But just how finely should we divide a construct?

There is a deceptively simple answer to this question: we should divide a construct into levels that make a clinically meaningful difference! As I said above, we want measures that are meaningfully sensitive to changes in the construct of interest. But of course, this answer only pushes our question back one step: How do we determine clinically meaningful difference? How do we know when the questions we ask in patient-centered measures are sufficiently fine-grained? How do we know if they are too fine-grained? In part, the answer to this latter question can be understood statistically. Questions that are considered too close to one another will have overlapping standard errors. Standard errors are a way of telling, from a statistical perspective, if one question is significantly different from another. If standard errors overlap, this tells us that two questions are similar enough to be indistinguishable.[1] But even if there are upper limits to how finely we can divvy up the questions in a measure, there is still latitude in their granulation. How do we know when our questions are addressing clinically meaningful difference? How do we know what is clinically meaningful? I argued in Chapter 3 that the kinds of questions we pose in a measure should be determined in large part though epistemic dialogue. If we want to know what makes for clinically meaningful differences, we should take care to listen to people with disabilities, patients, and other ill persons. I still think this is true, but it's now time to complicate my concept of epistemic dialogue.

In Chapter 3 I was concerned with making the point that those with firsthand experience with disability, disease, and illness have an epistemic and ethical role to play in the development of patient-centered measures. At the same time, I wanted to be clear that this role is not absolute: health researchers cannot abnegate their own epistemic and ethical responsibilities when they learn to respect those of others. Epistemic dialogue was introduced to bring first- and secondhand perspectives to bear on patient-centered constructs. But epistemic dialogue is not one and done; it is iterative across both measure development and the ongoing coordination of patient-centered measures. We might say epistemic dialogue characterizes patient-centered measures— its development, its application, its analysis. It's how we should conceptualize the back-and-forth of published materials, conference talks, seminar room discussions, and so on. Moreover, as one of its characteristics, the participants in epistemic dialogue should be wide-ranging—not only between people with disabilities, patients, and other ill persons, and health researchers, but also among different health researchers, between health researchers and philosophers, between health researchers and clinicians, and so on.

Increasingly questions about the responsiveness of patient-centered measures are presented as questions of scientific rigor (Hobart et al. 2007; Mokkink et al. 2019): For instance, as part of their argument for Rasch-based measures Hobart et al. (2007, 1095) write, "To our knowledge there are no published studies that show the scientific superiority of single item scales over multiple items scales." They assume, correctly I think, that their audience will be best persuaded by the Rasch measurement model's superiority if they can argue it is scientifically superior to its competitors. This rhetorical device serves to obscure the values, for instance, harms and benefits, that are employed when health researchers make decisions about sensitivity; it also obscures who stands to gain financially or otherwise from more sensitive measures. We might say it serves to limit the relevance relations we can bring to bear on questions of responsiveness in patient-centered measures, which in turn limits those who can take part in this dialogue. I want to argue that this is a mistake, that dialogue about the appropriate responsiveness of these measures is part of epistemic dialogue and as such should be open to a variety of interests (or relevance relations). One of the ways this emphasis on science plays out is through the use of latent trait measurement models over CTT measurement models. The idea is that latent trait models are more scientific than CTT ones. In what follows I use an example from Rasch to make my case that this emphasis on science is misplaced.

In Chapter 1 I argued that Rasch and CTT fail to coordinate patient-centered measures with the constructs they aim to assess. Nonetheless, Rasch is a scientific improvement on CTT because it is falsifiable and provides an ordering of questions with increasing difficulty on a linear scale; that is, it offers an improvement on interpretability. Rasch measurement theory says that people's response to a question is determined by the difference between their location on the ruler (how much ability they have) and a question's location on the ruler (how much ability a question requires). The Rasch scale runs from plus to minus infinity with the zero point at the place where the difficulty of the items in the survey is equal to the ability of the sample population. Each question is located on the ruler relative to the point at which there is equal probability of respondents answering yes or no to that question. Thus, what we get with Rasch is a ruler with items placed along it according to their difficulty.

The ordering that Rasch offers is useful. In Chapter 1 I discussed how this ordering renders patient-centered measures more interpretable than CTT measures. But the ordering has another benefit. It makes clear where a measure is less sensitive and where it is more sensitive: where questions are closer together, the measure is more sensitive than areas on the ruler where questions are farther apart. Moreover, if a ruler has more questions clustering around, say, the difficult end, then this measure is more sensitive to people with more ability. One of the arguments some make for using Rasch measures is to improve the likelihood that clinical trials will deliver effective treatments (Hobart et al. 2007). The idea is that perhaps clinical trials fail because our measures aren't very good at detecting benefit. If so, perhaps Rasch can help with this problem.

Imagine you are wondering if a particular candidate measure is appropriate to use in a clinical trial to establish the effectiveness of a drug. Imagine this candidate measure uses the Rasch measurement model. How do we decide if this candidate measure will do? We might consider using this measure to get the pretreatment scores of the population we hope will benefit. That is, we might look to see where the population's baseline scores are on the candidate measure. These scores can give us important information. If, for instance, baseline scores cluster at the difficult end of the ruler, then this measure may not be a good bet for our trial because our population may already have as much ability as this measure can assess; that is, this measure might not be sensitive to the benefits we hope to find. Alternatively, imagine the pretreatment scores tend to cluster at an area of the candidate measure that is insensitive, that is, where there are large gaps in questions. Here too we may think this isn't a very good measure for our trial because the drug would have to make a significant difference in ability for the candidate measure to pick it up. We might have reason to think the difference in ability the drug makes is small (albeit important). Or we might think it should make a big difference in ability, but we want to keep the stakes low given how much time and energy goes into clinical trials.

One response to this baseline clinical information is to create or update a measure, namely, one that is more sensitive. In the case where the pretreatment scores cluster at the difficult end of the ruler, we need to add questions to stretch out this part of the ruler. In the case where the pretreatment scores cluster at a part of the ruler that is relatively insensitive, we need to find questions that can fill out this part of the ruler. To be sure, researchers can't simply add questions willy-nilly. Rather, new questions need to be tested on the relevant population to determine their fit with the model, that is, the degree to which respondents' answers to the questions fit the predictions of the Rasch model within acceptable uncertainty.

This process of seeking to add questions is the opposite of what happened in the ABILHAND example I gave in Chapter 1. In that example questions were eliminated from the qualitative sample because they didn't fit the Rasch model, whereas in the current example we're looking to add questions that fit with the model. In Chapter 1 I criticized the ABILHAND for eliminating questions simply because they failed to fit the model. I argued instead this mismatch between the qualitative sample and the empirical item order should be a starting point for asking questions. Is there anything missing in the empirical ordering? Given what we know about manual ability in people with rheumatoid arthritis, does the empirical ordering teach us something new? What do people with rheumatoid arthritis think of the new ordering? In other words, the empirical item ordering should be a point for epistemic dialogue. Similarly, if we are going to add questions to an instrument to increase sensitivity, these alterations should also be a point for epistemic dialogue. Why are we adding these questions? How will a more sensitive measure benefit patients? How will it benefit pharmaceutical industries? Does the increase in sensitivity measure meaningful clinical difference? Why might these new questions not have arisen during the initial qualitative research? And so on.

Increasing the sensitivity or responsiveness of patient-centered measures is not simply a question of good science. It is also a question of values, for example, harms and benefits, and it is a question of business, for example, profits and losses. Questions that seek to illuminate these interests should be taken seriously if we want to avoid distortions that can subvert the integrity of science. For instance, those who voice concerns about type-1 errors, that is, the increase in false positive outcomes in a clinical trial that might result from more sensitive measures, should not be treated as scientifically or metrologically naive (Hobart et al. 2007). At the same time, we shouldn't assume that those who push for more responsive instruments are doing so merely out of an interest to attract the attention pharmaceutical industries. In other words, we shouldn't "pull rank" on those who ask these questions. Moreover, somewhat ironically, welcoming questions about type-1 errors and non-epistemic values such as harms and benefits is one way to demonstrate that one's interest in science is indeed genuine. This point is part of what I mean when I say we need to welcome interests in, for example, harms and benefits, and profits and losses, if we want to avoid distortions that can subvert the integrity of science.

Finally, sometimes questions about false positives or other concerns seen as tangential to the science of measurement are taken seriously, but put on hold, to be reserved for consideration at some later date once the "scientific" aspect of measurement design is over (Hobart et al. 2007). This is also a mistake. If, as I've been arguing in this book, patient-centered measures have the structure of a hermeneutic circle, then designing them and making them meaningful are processes that must go together. We develop our understanding of constructs and what makes for meaningful change as we measure—and as we listen to one another and continue to ask questions. This is not a tidy process where we first get the science correct and then we add in concerns about overtreatment or misuse. Rather, as I said in Chapter 1, measurement development is messy. This should remind us that in measurement as in much else we do not seek perfection. Rather we seek to do the very best with what we have at any given time. But to truly do our best we need to acknowledge the legitimacy of wide-ranging concerns; we need to take them seriously and assume we have something to learn.

6.1.2. Range and Targeting

When we think about range in the context of patient-centered measures, we talk about scale-to-sample targeting. Scale-to-sample targeting assesses the match between the range of a construct measured by a particular instrument and the range of the construct in the sample population. The idea is to ensure the questions on a measure can adequately address the ability of the population under measurement (Cleanthous et al. 2019). As with responsiveness, when targeting measures, clinical meaningfulness matters. Targeted measures should address only areas of a construct that make a clinically meaningful difference, so listening to people with disabilities, patients, and other ill persons is important when it comes to what parts of the construct should be measured. Focusing on parts of a construct that aren't important to patients—even if our measure has excellent sample-to-scale targeting—isn't an appropriate strategy for patient-centered measures. This point about the relationship between targeting and clinical significance is not controversial in the patient-centered measurement community.

Targeting is a part of good science, but it also involves questions of values, for instance, harms and benefits, and questions of business, for instance, profits, losses, and markets. Consider two examples, first a personal one. I recently had a hip replacement. Before my surgery I was asked to fill out a few patient-centered measures. The measures asked about my pain and mobility. There was a general pain scale; for example, rate your pain 1–10, and specific questions about how my pain limited my activities. There were also mobility questions that ranged from being able to dress oneself (low level of ability) to being able to run two miles (high level of ability). My average pain was about a 2 or a 3, but pain didn't limit any of the activities they listed, and I had as much mobility as they measured (I could run two miles). You might say that I hit the ceiling on both the activity and mobility measures. Given my answers, there are two different inferences we might make. We might infer that I didn't need a hip replacement. If I could still run and pain didn't limit my activities, then maybe my hip wasn't bad enough to warrant a replacement. Another way to think about this is to say getting a new hip wouldn't sufficiently improve my quality of life to warrant a replacement. Alternatively, we might infer the instruments I was measured on had poor scale-to-sample targeting; that is, the range of ability measured by these instruments was poorly matched to the ability in the sample population. Put differently, the measures couldn't assess higher levels of ability and mobility, and thus weren't sensitive to losses of ability toward the upper end of the scale. That is, the measures had ceiling effects.

Are ceiling effects in measurement bad? I sometimes live in Ireland and as my hip continued to bother me, I started to make my way through the rounds of consultations, referrals, and MRIs. But the Irish healthcare system didn't want to replace my hip. It turns out, the decision-makers were quite content with measurement ceiling effects. In fact, they use them as cutoff points for the upper end of ability where treatment is warranted. The Irish Health Service Executive (HSE 2020) website gives examples that might warrant hip replacement; the examples are almost identical to the questions I had to answer on the patient-centered measures:

- Severe pain, swelling and stiffness in your hip joint and reduced mobility.
- Pain so severe it interferes with your quality of life and sleep.
- Everyday tasks such as shopping or getting out of the bath are difficult or impossible.
- Feeling depressed because of the pain and lack of mobility.
- Can't work or have a normal social life.

As with the questions on the patient-centered measures, my hip problems didn't rise to the severity indicated here. Yet I was still very frustrated with my inability to do the things I wanted to do. I could run two miles, but I couldn't run it comfortably, and I couldn't run every day, nor could I run much more than two miles—things I had done regularly up until about five years ago. Plus, riding my horse had become increasingly difficult. I was crooked in the saddle, my balance in the stirrups was poor, and swinging my leg over to mount and dismount was hard. And (!) the leg attached to my bad hip was a good inch longer than my other leg, which caused pain in my back. It wasn't severe and didn't stop me from sleeping but I couldn't stand up properly or walk normally. So when I encountered these roadblocks in Ireland I traveled to the United States, where I also sometimes live. I found a top-notch surgeon (shout out to Dr. Otero), who cheerfully told me he could give me my life back with minimal pain and almost no rehabilitation. I took him up on it, and just like that, I'm riding and running like new. I can bend and twist and jump; I've stopped worrying that one of my kids will run into my leg. I'm less grumpy and more positive. It feels like a miracle. My quality of life is *much* improved.

What should we make of my new hip vis-à-vis scale-to-sample targeting? One thing I can say with certainty is from this patient's perspective, getting a new hip has vastly improved my quality of life. The upper levels of ability not measured by the patient-centered instruments I was given (ironically in the United States), clearly, to my mind, fail to measure levels of ability that can transform a person's life. So, from this first-person perspective, the ceiling effects are problematic cutoffs, and scale-to-sample targeting would not only benefit from better measurement of upper ability levels, but also justify the replacement of hips like mine. All of this said, when we think about scale-to-sample targeting, the first-person perspective is important, but it is only part of what we need to consider. Recall epistemic dialogue. It was introduced to address criticisms that people with disabilities, patients, and other ill persons points of view can distort our understanding of a construct or its clinical significance just as they can also enhance it. Epistemic dialogue says we can learn from firsthand experience, but we should not acquiesce to it. Rather we should question it; add to it. Thus, in addition to my first-person point of view that early hip replacement is beneficial, we need to widen our considerations to be confident in this view.

Better targeting of higher ability levels for hip replacements will likely increase the number of these interventions. Measuring at the higher ability end of the scale means replacing more hips on younger people. My hip feels great now, but to understand whether replacing hips on younger people is all things considered a good idea, we need more information. For instance, artificial hips don't last forever, so it's important to know when a population will need a revision and the likely outcomes for this procedure on a younger population who will likely need more revisions. Moreover, in many healthcare systems the associated cost of replacing hips on younger people and the associated revisions must be considered against other resource needs in the same system. Quality Adjusted Life Years (QALYs) are typically used by health systems to both value and compare health outcomes. Moreover, using QALY data and information on the costs associated with early versus delayed hip replacements can provide information on the cost per QALY to a health-care system (e.g., Mota 2013). Because QALYs and costs can vary, the decision of when hip replacements are warranted—and thus when ceiling effects are justified—will vary from country to country.

Now consider a less personal example. In their article "The ADAS-cog in Alzheimer's Disease Clinical Trials: Psychometric Evaluation of the Sum and Its Parts," Stefan Cano and colleagues (2010) evaluate the Alzheimer's Disease Assessment Scale Cognitive Behavior Section (ADAS-cog) for targeting issues. The ADAS-cog is a widely used primary outcome measure in clinical trials for Alzheimer's Disease.[2] It measures 11 components such as word recall, word recognition, word finding, and naming objects and fingers. In their study, Cano and colleagues investigated the scale-to-sample findings of each of these components. They found significant ceiling effects in over half the components in the ADAS-cog, with more than 75% of participants scoring a 0 or 1 in these areas (a score of zero suggests no problems with cognitive ability and a score of 1 suggests few problems). These results suggest to the authors ceiling effects in the respective components because, as in any population—even those at the upper end of the ability scale—we would expect to see clinical heterogeneity in the study population. Instead, in these components we see over three-quarters of participants clumped at one end of the scale. Another way to put this point is to say the cognitive limitations of this population don't seem to be well matched to the range of the ADAS-cog.

For the authors, the upshot of this mismatch is that clinical trials may fail to identify differences. Poorly targeted measures are likely to underestimate changes over time and differences between groups for some populations. Since clinical trials in Alzheimer's disease and other forms of dementia are "tending to recruit people with milder Alzheimer's disease" (Cano et al. 2010, 1366), ceiling effects in measures such as the ADAS-cog would seem to subvert the purpose of these trials; that is, they would seem to subvert finding differences and change over time in a high-cognitive-ability Alzheimer's population. As our understanding of Alzheimer's disease improves, so do our efforts to produce treatments that will slow down (or alter) the course of the disease earlier in its progression. If Cano and colleagues are correct about the ceiling effects of the ADAS-cog, then this instrument may not be able to detect the clinical benefits of the latest pharmaceutical candidates. Cano and his colleagues imply that this inability is a bad thing, and we probably don't need a qualitative study or public meeting to know that people with early Alzheimer's disease and those who care for them would agree. In fact, my grandmother died from complications from Alzheimer's disease after a long and grim existence with it. If this is something I inherit, then I want drugs that slow the disease progression to a standstill as early as possible. I want measures that can detect group differences and change over time in populations with high-cognitive-ability Alzheimer's disease.

Imagine, for the sake of argument, that after epistemic dialogue we agree with this initial first-person perspective: we ought to target the components of the ADAS-cog to the high-cognitive-ability Alzheimer's disease population. This decision will hopefully increase the chances of a successful clinical trial that will advance our ability to manage Alzheimer's disease better and earlier. But there will be other likely effects of these measures. More people will be diagnosed with Alzheimer's disease earlier, possibly without treatment to help them, at least for now; drugs might be discovered, but they may be out of reach financially for many people; drugs may be discovered but their effectiveness might be small; the approved drugs may have serious side effects that in turn need to be managed. My point here is that even if, after epistemic dialogue, targeting the ADAS-cog is deemed beneficial, there are likely to be associated harms as well. Thus, we shouldn't think about scale-to-sample targeting as an unmitigated good, as Cano and colleagues (2010) seem to do. In their article, the benefits of scale-to-sample targeting are tied to improving the success of clinical trials. And while positive clinical trials are *sometimes* in the best interest of people with disabilities, patients, and other ill persons, they are *always* in the best interest of pharmaceutical and medical device companies. Clinical research is important, but it would be naive to ignore the financial stakes involved in a successful trial. Given this fact, when we consider targeting a measure to a specific population, we should be alive to the harms as well as benefits and the financial stakes some may have in promoting measurement changes. To improve the likelihood that epistemic dialogue will address these harms, it is important to include different perspectives, especially those who are likely to disagree with mainstream views. Indeed, as I discussed in Chapter 3, engaging with perspectives different from our own or what is mainstream is essential for epistemic dialogue to be able to put our own assumptions and values into relief.

6.2. Industry's Influence beyond Measurement

Pharmaceutical companies make money when they sell drugs to more people in diverse markets. Measurement is one tool these companies can use to expand their presence in these markets. There is a saying that "what gets measured gets managed." As I discussed above, creating more responsive and targeted measures increases the number of people who get managed because it increases the evidence we have to marshal arguments for treatment. In medicine, management often means treatment, and treatment, although it can mean many things—hope, despair, excitement, dread—also typically means money, money that flows out of some coffers and into others.

Nonetheless, as I also discuss above, we can't simply stretch out a portion of a patient-centered measure or target any old population; that is, we can't try to manage just any population. One of the conditions for patient-centered measures is clinical meaningfulness. In this context that means we need some evidence that greater responsiveness or targeting is warranted from the perspectives of people with disabilities, patients, and other ill persons. Yet as Holman and Geisler (2018) show, when the stakes are high, patient perspectives can be purchased. Even so, in the section above I suggest the solution to—let's just call it what it is—corrupt measurement is epistemic dialogue. But how can that be the solution when relations of power (and power is everywhere, thank you Foucault, e.g., 1963/1973 and 1975/1977) risk the distortion of dialogue? In the final section of this chapter, I will address this question. In this section, I want to continue to worry you about the opportunities that exist for pharmaceutical and medical device companies to measure what matters *to them*. In the previous section I explored how measure development and design can feed into a financial bottom line. In this section I zoom out one step to look at the opportunities drug and medical device companies have to use their influence in clinical research and medical communication more generally.

Influence is an important word when we talk of pharmaceutical industries and medical knowledge. As Sergio Sismondo argues in his book *Ghost-Managed Medicine Big Pharma's Invisible Hands* (2018), the concern we ought to have about industry's involvement in medical knowledge is not primarily one about false or unjustified knowledge claims; the problem is not necessarily bad science.[3] Rather the concern is *influence* over the construction of medical knowledge at almost every decision point—pharmaceutical industries sponsor roughly half of all clinical trials, produce a significant portion of the medical literature, create and manage key opinion leaders to help market their products through education and conference presentations, and fund two-thirds of all patient advocacy organizations (Sismondo 2018). Indeed, Sismondo writes that around 93% of patient advocacy organizations that make presentations to the FDA receive industry funding (the example of flibanserin was not a one-off). Pharmaceutical industries produce, distribute, and encourage the consumption of their medical knowledge. And the problem with their nearly ubiquitous presence is the way their interests *influence* the shape of medical knowledge over time, not with the methods of their science.

Industry-funded research produces knowledge that favors industry products, knowledge that increases market share. When the products are primarily drugs, the result is that we are sicker through expanded disease categories and through side effects of drugs. Sismondo (2018, 180) writes:

To increase their markets, pharma-sponsored medical studies and guidelines tend to expand the definitions and prominence of specific diseases. This increases the number of people potentially affected. Pharma's selective but aggressive distribution of medical information promotes symptoms and diagnoses to physicians and patients. Patients present themselves to their doctors with complaints shaped by pharma promotion and readily available pharma-sponsored information. Physicians may then understand their patients, and patients may understand themselves, in terms laid out by the industry.

Earlier I said that an emphasis on the scientific rigor in measurement design can obscure the values employed when health researchers make decisions about, for example, sensitivity or range; it also obscures who stands to gain financially or otherwise from more sensitive or targeted measures. Sismondo (2018) makes a similar point when discussing industry's involvement in producing articles for medical journals. Editors of medical journals rely on author guidelines and standardized rules that govern the performance and analysis of clinical trials to control for bias and ensure high-quality medical science. Industry-funded trials typically score well on methodological tests. In fact, Sismondo (2018, 89–90) argues that industry-managed science looks very much like independent science; he even goes so far as to say it looks particularly clean and successful in comparison. We might translate this as saying that industry science looks particularly well justified; that is, it looks exceptionally scientific. Recall from Chapter 4 that, when discussing standardized questions, I argued they are conceptualized as aiding mechanical objectivity (Daston and Gailson 2007; Reiss 2020). Mechanical objectivity seeks to reduce interpretation and replace it with procedures that "move nature to the page." It isn't only standardized questions that are ostensibly used to boost objectivity: publishing guidelines, rules, and methods seek to do the same. Yet, Sismondo argues, rather than ensure the publication of objective science, the rules and guidelines that frame publication practically serve to distance the relevant parties—publishers, editors, authors, industry—from responsibility for the bias that pervades industry-curated articles. Science, understood as a collection of methods, rules, standardized metrics, and procedures is used as a cloaking device that makes questions about values and interests appear irrelevant and unscientific.

Sismondo is not the only one to make this kind of point. Bennet Holman (2019) argues similarly, but his target is mainstream philosophy of medicine, which, he argues, tends to focus on "friction-free epistemology." Friction-free epistemology examines ideal experimentation and abstracts away from real-world details in order to understand the underlying logical structure of inference. Friction-free epistemology is representative of a way of thinking that separates philosophy of science from sociology of science, that is, the study of logic and inference from the study of human interactions. The problem with friction-free epistemology is not that it isn't appropriate in some circumstances, but it isn't appropriate in all circumstances—even philosophical ones. For instance, if we are trying to answer a question in principle, then friction-free epistemology is a good strategy since the actual details aren't relevant. But philosophers, particularly philosophers of medicine, often take themselves to be answering questions about non-idealized situations about what actual doctors/regulators/patients should do with actual evidence. In cases where philosophers address non-idealized circumstances, their analysis must include the relevant messy details to escape drawing the wrong epistemic conclusions. Holman (2019) argues that philosophers must take into account industry funding and commercial imperatives if they are to develop a credible account of medical knowledge.

To illustrate the problem with friction-free epistemology, Holman (2019) develops an example of class-I antiarrhythmic drugs used to suppress ventricle extra beats (VEBs) and, supposedly, cardiac death. But it turns out that using these drugs to suppress VEBs increases cardiac death, a fact that was only discovered during a National Institutes for Health–sponsored randomized controlled trial. Philosophers have used this example to argue for the superiority of statistical, that is, evidence-based medicine, over causal reasoning in medicine. Holman (2019) argues that philosophers have missed the point. The problem with the use of antiarrhythmic drugs wasn't poor logical inference, but rather a decision about what to measure. The decision was made to measure the efficacy of these drugs in terms of their ability to suppress VEBs rather than their ability to lower mortality rates. This decision benefited pharmaceutical industries and was, on Holman's telling, influenced by them. Indeed, Holman relates the details of a conference organized by these industries in the early 1980s in which industry representatives, academic researchers, and members of the FDA met to discuss what evidence the FDA would accept to establish the efficacy of antiarrhythmic drugs. The point of the conference was to establish guidelines. Pharmaceutical industries lobbied for the suppression of VEBs to be used as a surrogate endpoint instead of the clinical endpoint of mortality. They argued that cardiac death as an endpoint was prohibitively expensive, whereas the evidence on VEBs suppression was available and analyzable. The FDA eventually agreed.

Holman (2019) concludes when we ignore the source of evidence and focus only on the science (FDA) or idealized conditions (philosophy), we risk making epistemic mistakes. Indeed, he concludes that industry funding is part of scientific experimentation just as study design and logical inference are a part of it. Economic and commercial interests affect the questions that get asked and the methods and measures used. We cannot afford to ignore them. Yet ignorance is widespread. Consider an example from patient-centered measurement.

Hobart et al. (2007) have argued that patient-centered measures are difficult to interpret and have questionable sensitivity and targeting. They suggest these limitations could be an impediment to accurate estimates of effect size and detection of clinical change. Moreover, they submit that failures of clinical trials to yield larger numbers of effective treatments may be due to the lack of scientific rigor of the measuring instruments used in these trials. It shouldn't be surprising that pharmaceutical companies looking for ways to maximize the success of their clinical trials to get their product to market will be interested in securing measures that might further their goal. But it's not only pharmaceutical industries that want to see the acceleration of medical product development. The FDA also shares this goal, albeit for different reasons. If pharmaceutical industries want to make drugs available to the public to increase profits, the FDA wants to make drugs available to enhance public health. They share an interest in the public's access to drugs and medical devices, but their motivations differ.

FDA guidelines are one way that rules of engagement for this shared interest are spelled out.[4] In the FDA's (2009) "Patient-Reported Outcome Measures: Use in Medical Product Development to Support Labeling Claims" scientific rigor and clinical significance are the lingua franca of engagement. Thus, if more sensitive and targeted measures can be packaged as meeting the FDA's scientific standards to a higher degree while also better serving patients, it's a win-win for everyone. Medical device and pharmaceutical industries get measuring instruments that may increase the likelihood of successful clinical trials and greater market access; the FDA increases the likelihood that labeling claims on new drugs and devices reflect our best measurement science regarding subjective health. The scientific thresholds having been passed, questions about values and profits seem beside the point if not a bit gauche. Afterall, the FDA's mission is limited, and preventing medical device and pharmaceutical industries from making a profit is not part of it.

Patient-centered measures function as a node within industry's expansive web of influence, but if so, how does this happen, practically speaking? What is the institutional infrastructure that brings measurement design into these industries' orbit? I have mentioned Holman's discussion of an industry-sponsored conference that brought industry representative, academic researchers, and members of the FDA together to discuss guidelines. There are now formal, precompetitive spaces that have been developed that enable these same parties to come together to work out what measures and methods might meet everyone's needs. For example, public-private partnerships, such as Critical Path Institute (C-Path) created in 2005 under the auspices of the FDA's critical path initiative program, aim to create drug development tools (DDTs). DDTs include new data, measurement, and method standards to accelerate the pace and reduce the cost of medical product development (Critical Path Institute 2015). C-Path puts industry scientists and academic consultants together to develop tools that will enhance the ability of medical device and pharmaceutical industries to develop medical products. The FDA then provides iterative feedback on the tools they create, hopefully ending in the approval of the DDT for use in specific product development. Patient-reported outcomes are one of the four types of clinical outcome assessments eligible to qualify as a DDT (FDA 2022b).

Partly through the work of Sismondo, the philosophical and bioethics community has learned to have a healthy skepticism about industry-academic partnerships (McClimans 2017). Much of Sismondo's work focuses on publication ethics through "ghost-managed" research (Sismondo 2018; Sismondo and Doucet 2010; Sismondo and Nicholson 2009; Sismondo 2007). Sismondo writes that in some high-profile medical journals nearly 40% of published articles on recently approved drugs are ghost-managed by pharmaceutical industries (Sismondo 2018, 15). The ghostly nature of this management is reflected in their largely invisible hand in the process. Sismondo (2018, 66) describes the ghostly work of publication planners who take the scientific and commercial value out of clinical study data and analyses to construct articles that establish consistent profiles for drugs. Pharmaceutical industry statisticians and professional medical writers author the articles, but, Sismondo argues, the articles are published under the names of academic researchers. These academic researchers may sit on an advisory board for a pharmaceutical company or supply patients for their study; they researchers may edit the paper or merely sign off on it. But whatever their relationship to the article, it isn't the kind we typically imagine, where researchers design and run studies, extract data, run analyses, and then write up their findings.

Sismondo identifies the entangled nature of these curated publications as practically expedient, but epistemically and ethically troubling. It is practically expedient because everyone seems to win: pharmaceutical industries get more market value out of their publications if well-respected researchers put their names on the manuscripts; researchers get publications in notable journals; journals get well-cited manuscripts, which if published will produce revenue in the form of offprints purchased by industry (Sismondo and Doucet 2010). The troubling aspect of this process is to my mind the consistent orientation of these articles toward a positive message of more drugs for more people. The problem isn't so much that industry's science is flawed, but rather the questions they are interested in answering shape our body of medical knowledge in a biased manner. For instance, through pharmaceutical industry activity we learn a lot about what happens on the margins of health rather than in the middle of it (to use Sismondo's [2018] phrase). We learn, for instance, about marginally effective drugs that open markets in new populations. The upshot is more people are categorized as sick, and more people are taking marginally effective drugs. More people on more drugs means more people experiencing harmful side effects.

I'm not suggesting here that precompetitive spaces such as C-Path necessarily lead to the same kind of ethical questions industry-curated publications do. At the same time, I am suggesting that the language of science and clinical meaningfulness are not enough to safeguard DDTs from bias. Pharmaceutical industry representatives have an explicit agenda, and for academic consultants, measurement development can be a lucrative side hustle. Indeed, for some it turns into a full-time job when they realize they can make more consulting for the pharmaceutical industry than they can working for the public good at a university. I want to be clear: academic consultants are not the "bad guys" in this story, and neither are industry representatives. Industry representatives have a job to do, and C-Path and other such spaces offer an opportunity to do it well. Moreover, when academic consultants find their skills sought after and valued, they aren't to blame when they work for the pharmaceutical industry. The problem is not individuals, but I do think part of the problem is the narrow rules of engagement that allow biased measures and scientific knowledge to proliferate under the banner of scientific rigor.

Throughout this chapter I've discussed scientific rigor and clinical meaningfulness as if they were two distinct concepts. But clinical meaningfulness is also subsumed under the category of scientific rigor. Recall earlier I mentioned some of the methodological approaches to establishing clinical significance for interpretability in distribution and anchor-based approaches, or combinations of the two. Moreover, in Chapter 3 I discussed how the FDA guidelines for the use of patient-centered measures in labeling claims understood representing patients' voices in terms of qualitative research. Whether clinical meaningfulness refers to interpretability or measure development, health researchers and others tend to think about it in the narrow terms of scientific rigor. I have argued in this book and elsewhere (McClimans 2011) that this approach is misguided. Science is wonderful, but if we are going to succeed in revealing even some of the biases that come from individual and corporate interests, then we need something more, and that more is epistemic dialogue.

But how is epistemic dialogue going to help reveal unwanted bias when the very actors we depend upon to provide perspectives, and to ask and answer questions about disability and illness, can be co-opted by ideology and powerful interests? Before I answer this question, I want to end this section with a personal story. A few years ago, I was approached to be a coauthor on an article criticizing a particular measure. I was offered what seemed to me a large sum of money to write about something I agree is problematic. I wanted to go on a summer holiday with my family that year, so, for financial reasons, I was tempted to agree to the invitation. But the organization behind the offer was a patient advocacy group sponsored by industry. I tell this story to both emphasize how expansive industry's influence extends, and to illustrate the ease with which one can become caught up in its influence. I would've been writing about a methodological, and in fact ethical, problem I believe exists with this measure, and I would have gotten a publication and a holiday out of it. But it was an article I never would have considered writing on my own and submitted to a journal not of my own choosing, and it would have been used as a mean to ends I couldn't control, but could possibly foresee.

6.3. Pulling Rank and Epistemic Dialogue

As the previous section hopefully made clear, pharmaceutical industry's influence over drugs extends far and wide. Pharmaceutical industries don't simply develop new drugs and manufacture existing ones, they also fund research, develop measures and methods, curate journal articles, partner with academic researchers, lobby the FDA, and market their products. Within this vast array of activity there are numerous places where they can bias production, evaluation, and dissemination of information (Holman and Elliot 2018). As public trust of industry-sponsored research wanes, it's important to be clear that the industry's involvement in research is not purely negative. Many valuable products come to market through industry dollars (Besley et al. 2017). Yet even if pharmaceutical industry's involvement was purely problematic, it is so entrenched in producing, evaluating, and disseminating research that eliminating its influence is unrealistic. It thus behooves us to find ways to limit those deleterious assumptions and values that accompany industry sponsorship while supporting those that promote knowledge.

While in the previous section I cast a wide net to illustrate the extensive scope of the pharmaceutical industry's influence, in this section I return to the question of epistemic dialogue as a mechanism of clinical meaningfulness. Epistemic dialogue, as I discuss in Chapter 3, can be understood as a form of critical dialogue oriented toward achieving a better—more coherent or impactful—understanding of a topic through the give-and-take of questions and answers. It's through this give-and-take that prejudice and bias that present obstacles to better understandings are uncovered and shed, while those that enhance our understanding are clarified. I am not the first to suggest a form of critical dialogue as a strategy for uncovering prejudice and bias. Indeed, in the philosophical literature it is one of the leading suggestions for improving the quality of pharmaceutical industry-sponsored research and policy decision-making. For instance, as I discuss in Chapter 3, Bueter and Jukola (2020) argue that the public meeting on flibanserin may have had a different outcome if participants were encouraged to respond to arguments made by other discussants. As they argue, critical discourse may safeguard against bias. Similarly, Kevin Elliot (2018) has argued that effective criticism might be used to establish the objectivity of scientific research, which in turn can be used as a criterion to evaluate and improve the quality of industry-funded research. His suggestion follows from work on scientific objectivity from philosophers such as Heather Douglas (2004, 2009), Sandra Harding (2015), Elizabeth Lloyd (1995), and Helen Longino (1990, 2002). The goal of effective criticism as Elliot thinks about it is to uncover and evaluate the implicit assumptions that shape the choice of methods and measures, as well as interpretations of research findings.

In describing effective criticism, Elliot relies on Longino's (1990, 2002) characterization of objective science as "contextual empiricism." For criticism to be effective in improving objectivity, contextual empiricism calls for publicly recognized venues for criticism, uptake of criticism, shared standards, and the tempered equality of intellectual authority. Consider the need to have venues where critical dialogue can take place. When we think about pharmaceutical industry-funded research done for the purposes of regulation, for instance, drug approval, then agencies such as the FDA are prime candidates to serve as venues for criticism—and indeed the FDA does engage in this activity. For example, the FDA convenes multidisciplinary advisory committees and panels to provide independent expert advice on scientific, technical, and policy matters (FDA, n.d.). This advice can be understood as a form of effective criticism. Moreover, as I discussed in Chapter 3, from 2012 to 2017 the FDA hosted 24 disease-specific patient-focused drug development meetings to obtain information about specific diseases and treatments from patients' perspectives. These meetings also can serve as a venue for effective criticism. To be sure there are potential and actual problems with these venues if, for instance, meetings are "captured" (Holman and Geisler 2018; Biddle 2013) or if, to take another example, the questions the FDA asks its multidisciplinary advisory to discuss are overly narrow. Nonetheless, these venues exist as sites under the auspices of the FDA where effective criticism of drug applications can take place.

Justin Biddle (2013) has argued for a new venue to be established within the FDA, one that would institutionalize dissent and criticism. He develops an idea presented by Arthur Kantrowitz (1967) to establish a "science court" where scientific questions relevant to policy decisions would be adjudicated. The reason for this court, as Biddle relates, was to provide an institutional setting where decisions that are a mix of scientific, moral, and policy concerns could be addressed. The idea was to have two groups, one advocating for a position and the other against it, with a third party, a judge, presiding. As Biddle (2013) discusses, Kantrowitz thought such a system could eliminate prejudice and bias from policymaking and force scientists on opposing sides to engage in policy disputes in ethically and epistemically appropriate ways.

Biddle adopts this idea and applies it to the FDA as a way to evaluate and improve industry-funded drug applications. He calls his proposal the Adversarial Proceedings for the Evaluation of Pharmaceuticals. As Kantrowitz envisioned, Biddle imagines pharmaceutical representatives arguing explicitly for the safety and efficaciousness of a drug, while another group would take the case against it, and a third group would adjudicate the case. To my mind, the most interesting and promising aspect of Biddle's suggestion is that participants in this process couldn't be viewed as disinterested parties. By forcing groups to take a side—for or against approval—the decision-making process would presuppose a vested interest, which would illuminate the kinds of questions I suggest in Section 6.2 are currently lacking: questions of values and questions of economics. Put differently, decisions to approve a drug for public use would no longer be framed narrowly as a matter of scientific rigor presented by parties disinterested by the outcome.

Are proposals for epistemic dialogue or effective criticism or even science courts naive? Holman and Geisler (2018) suggest the answer is, perhaps, yes. The problem with these proposals is they explicitly require or tacitly presuppose that each contribution to the dialogue, criticism, or case have equal weight. That is, as we strive to understand better what quality of life with epilepsy is or what is quality of life with FSD, we consider each party to the dialogue as having equal epistemic and ethical worth. We don't discount testimony in advance because it comes from, say, a woman or an industry representative. We don't pull rank. Even science courts that would eventually decide in favor of one party's argument over another, shouldn't begin with prejudice. Indeed, this idea of equality is made explicit in the fourth characteristic of Longino's objective science, on which Elliot relies for his account of effective criticism: tempered equality of intellectual authority. Yet Holman and Geisler (2018) argue that in the case of industry-funded research, this presumption of equality is precisely what allows pharmaceutical industries to "crowd out the opposition." And they aren't alone. Within contemporary philosophy of science Manuela Fenández Pinto (2014) has argued similarly. Moreover, as I mention at the beginning of this chapter, feminists and other philosophers such as Habermas have worried about how relations of power and self-interest can distort expressions of need and value while misdirecting goals (Warnke 2014). If we take all comers seriously as possibly shedding light on a topic, then we risk perpetuating and codifying interests that seek profit and self-aggrandizement rather than truth.

This worry about codifying the wrong interests or having the wrong interests crowd out more socially valuable interests is clarified in Holman's (2015) and Holman and Geisler's (2018) work characterizing the relationship between industry and the FDA as an asymmetric arms race. The idea, as you may imagine, is one where the reliability of a strategy, say the use of patient-focused meetings to increase the relevance of drug development, decreases over time. In other words, over time patient-focused meetings will lose their ability to increase the real-world relevance of drug development. This loss in reliability occurs because pharmaceutical industries seek to exploit the weakness of any strategy that might prove an obstacle to drug development and approval. The FDA in turn responds to this exploitation with mechanisms that aim to shore up the discovered weakness. Mechanisms to circumvent exploitation are costly, so they are unlikely to be implemented until pharmaceutical industries make them necessary. Yet as is the nature of an arms race, once counter-mechanisms are implemented, these industries will simply seek to exploit further weaknesses. This process continues with the gradual accumulation of increasingly costly and often cumbersome mechanisms in response to relations of power and self-interest.

Holman and Geisler (2018) suggest three morals follow from their analogy. First, strategies employed within an asymmetric arms race aren't durable. If patient involvement is a good way to improve the relevance of drug development and approval, then we shouldn't expect it to remain a good strategy for long—at least to the degree this strategy runs counter to powerful interests such as industry. And following on from this idea is a second moral: strategies are more durable when they align epistemically and financially with the incentives driving an interaction. Finally, the third moral: strategies must do more than address current problems, they must anticipate and adjust for them. Thus, Holman and Geisler argue, agencies such as the FDA should work up robust solutions that anticipate countermoves before pharmaceutical industry's actions make them necessary. In the case of flibanserin, they suggest prohibiting participants with conflicts of interest such as industry affiliation.

Holman and Geisler's morals are less instructions for how to avoid an asymmetric arms race than they are how to become better at the game: recognize you're in an arms race, try to align incentives, and be prepared to increase the staying power of your strategy by thinking like the opposition. Getting better, in this context, means perpetuating relations of power. In the context of the flibanserin meetings, limiting participants to those without conflicts of interest would not stop industry from exerting influence (according to the arms race analogy, they would eventually find another way), but it would pull rank on whose testimony it denies. So much the better, some might say. When pharmaceutical industries take advantage of patient-focused public meetings, they essentially do the same. By flooding the meeting with industry-friendly patients and patient representatives, they dilute the testimony coming out of the meeting until what we learn reflects their interests, not everyday patients'.

Another way to analyze the pharmaceutical industry's behavior in the case of the flibanserin meeting is to think of it as breaking with the norms of scientific research, and in so doing, playing the FDA and perhaps the rest of us for fools. In Manuela Fernández Pinto's (2014) criticism of Longino's contextual empiricism, she argues along these lines. She suggests that the pillars of contextual empiricism, which Elliot relies on above to justify his effective criticism, are losing their normative force as new forms of engagement are developed out of the privatization and commercialization of scientific research. Where venues of criticism are supposed to promote public scrutiny of knowledge and limit the uptake of idiosyncratic values, Fernández Pinto points to the privatization of public venues that circumvent this intention. She gives the example of private peer review companies who charge a fee for peer review, thus limiting the kinds of authors who can avail themselves of this service. She also cites Sismondo's (2007, 2009) work on ghostwriting and publication planning. Along with these examples we might add strategies to flood public meetings with perspectives that skew the totality of what is expressed. In these examples, private companies officially play by the rules of science (and the law) but disregard the norms that governed them—norms such as truth, fruitfulness, coherence, and transparency. What should we do when there is a breakdown of the norms that guide practice? Or, as Richard Bernstein asked in the 1982 *Proceedings of the Biennial Meeting of the Philosophy of Science Association,*

What happens when there is a breakdown of such principles, when they no longer seem to have any normative power, when there are deep and apparently irreconcilable conflicts about such principles, or when questions are raised about the very norms and principles that ought to guide our praxis? (341)

Bernstein raises this question against the backdrop of a discussion of Gadamerian hermeneutics and Habermasian rationalism. He argues that both philosophers were concerned with these questions, just as Fernández Pinto is concerned. He thus suggests that the worry is not new—it is not a worry that comes with new trends in privatization and commercialization—but rather an older concern. To reiterate and generalize, the worry is that the ability for epistemic or critical dialogue to effectively guide science or even coordinate general human action is contingent on the existence of shared norms. The relevant norms may differ for guiding science than for coordinating human action, but what is important is they are shared and "inform the life of a community" (Bernstein 1982, 341). But when there is breakdown of shared norms, then, so goes the worry, epistemic or critical dialogue is no longer effective on its own.

Habermas puts the problem well when he writes that social (and I would also suggest scientific) institutions depend on language as a vehicle of organization and communication. Put differently, language is the medium of epistemic dialogue. But language also has another function: it is a medium of domination and social power, and "it serves to legitimate relations of organized force" (Habermas 1977, 360). In cases where shared norms are no longer applicable, where domination and social power work "behind the back of language" (Habermas 1977, 361) to affect the way we interpret, for instances, FSD, then, the worry continues, we need to do something else besides epistemic dialogue to get things done—to get science done, to coordinate human action. As Holman and Geisler (2018) suggest, maybe we need to become better at creating strategies that will be robust under conditions of an asymmetric arms race. Indeed, Fernández Pinto suggests philosophers of science need new norms, ones that are closer to the reality of privatized and commercial science than are the norms inherent in contextual empiricism; maybe one of these norms could be guided by the arms race analogy.

On the other hand, perhaps the answer to the arms race is not to perpetuate power, not to get better at the game. Perhaps the answer is to renounce epistemic power relations (Warnke 2014), to double down on epistemic dialogue. Epistemic dialogue, as a form of hermeneutic activity, fully embraces the recognition that every interpretation, every stab at knowledge, is incomplete. As humans we are temporally limited; we can never see the whole of that which we aim to understand. In his review of *Truth and Method*, Habermas (1977, 346) quotes Arthur Danto (1965, 142), who writes, "Completely to describe an event is to locate it in all the right stories, and this we cannot do. We cannot because we are temporally provincial with regard to the future." This limitation, which we cannot overcome, means that we will make mistakes in our interpretations and knowledge claims. We will sometimes project onto the topic of our inquiry false assumptions and inappropriate values, and because the whole is always out of reach, some of these false assumptions and values will stick longer than we would hope. Put differently, in the interplay between part and whole, between our tradition and the future, we sometimes have to wait longer than we would like for the future to correct the misconceptions of the past. This is simply to say that we are fallible and our knowledge claims are fallible.

But it is also to say that there is hope. It is to say that within the messiness of a past that includes the riches and misconceptions of all who have gone before us, we have the ability to move forward and correct what is wrong, to add to what is missing. But this ability to move forward is, at least for Gadamer, intimately tethered not only to coherence between part and whole, but also to an openness to learning—to epistemic humility. For Gadamer, our knowledge can only progress if we are willing and ready to learn something new, if we are willing to see in the whole, in the future, what we didn't see in the past. And this means that while we present what we know in the present with the confidence that comes from due diligence, we also must be ready to be wrong, for things to change. Fortitude is the sister of humility.

Yet sometimes when we get things wrong, when things change, there are serious and negative consequences—people are harmed, embarrassed, betrayed, made insecure; opportunities are lost; institutions fail; cultures can wither. Epistemic humility can seem an epistemic risk: What if we learn from the wrong things? What if we take patients and patient representatives seriously as authorities on FSD only to learn some of their testimony was planted? The piecemeal process of progress through fitting parts to whole, past to future, seems messy and uncertain—too messy, too uncertain. Perhaps we've learned enough. Perhaps we've learned enough to know what we don't want to learn.

At times we face an essential epistemic choice: embrace epistemic dialogue in full recognition of its limitations, or pull rank and decide from what and where we will learn. Both choices are risky. As I discuss above, we might learn the wrong things from the wrong people; we might be fooled, or we might fool ourselves. Either way, epistemic dialogue is fallible. On the other hand, pulling rank means deciding in advance that there is nothing to learn from someone or something. It also means using epistemic power to marginalize. History is littered with examples of pulling rank. Indeed, some of our greatest social problems are the result of pulling rank on whole swaths of a population, Irish people, Black people, Brown people, women of all identities. The resulting social problems help us to see that when we pull rank, we don't simply risk an opportunity to learn, we also reflect ourselves out of our relationship with others to objectify or patronize them (Warnke 2014). This power move perpetuates other power moves, much like the arms race described by Holman and Geisler (2018). This process continues with the gradual accumulation of increasingly costly and often cumbersome mechanisms that further entrench distrust and a lack of shared norms. Moreover, arms races quickly take on a life of their own. They may start out as a means to protect the integrity of knowledge or national sovereignty, but they often become a matter of staying in the game.

Tempting as it sometimes is, pulling rank is not a positive epistemic strategy. First, we are often wrong about what and where we can learn. Second, perpetuating epistemic power relations entrenches the instability of shared norms, and, third, it divides our epistemic pursuits. Rather than focusing on a topic of inquiry, our time and attention are diverted to enhancing the robustness of our strategies to block the opposition's attempts at exploitation. We end up learning the wrong things. But if pulling rank isn't the appropriate response to industry's capture of the FSD meeting, then what is? My suggestion is to double down on epistemic dialogue. When industry responds to patient-focused public meetings with a power move to capture them, the response should set aside the impulse to answer with epistemic power. Rather we—the FDA, the FDA's multidisciplinary advisory committee, other patients, and patient representatives—must be ready to take participants seriously and ask questions to understand better what FSD is. These questions should be wide-ranging to include questions about sponsorship and its effect on testimony. But nonetheless, they should be oriented toward building a coherent and impactful understanding that does justice to aspects of the case that are surprising or unusual, rather than oriented toward justification for dismissing some testimonies and highlighting others. They should be oriented toward an impactful if not shared understanding, keeping in mind that even when participants are sponsored by pharmaceutical industries, they are still people from whom we can learn and who can learn from us and, in fact, be transformed through dialogue (Warnke 2011).

Gadamer (2004, 371) writes in *Truth and Method*, "Among the greatest insights that Plato's account of Socrates affords us is that, contrary to the general opinion, it is more difficult to ask questions that to answer them." Epistemic dialogue is hard. While it has become fashionable in philosophy to talk of dialogue or effective criticism, it is not an easy skill to master. There is no method to asking questions; no method to learn what is questionable. Questioners must have knowledge of a topic, but also knowledge of what they don't know about it. They must be open to learning, toward revisiting previous assumptions. They must be tenacious and patient in the face of a dialogue that goes off the rails, for instance, due to cross purposes or a power play. They must be willing to keep asking questions. So, I say again: epistemic dialogue is hard, both from the perspective of a skill to be acquired and from the perspective of a virtue to hone. In fact, it is sufficiently difficult that if we had a better way forward, we would choose it. And yet, I submit, we do not have a better way.

6.4. Conclusion

Pharmaceutical industries have a vast influence over the production, evaluation, and dissemination of medical information. In this chapter I argue that this influence extends from the capture of the FDA meeting on FSD to the development of patient-centered measures. Nonetheless, if our epistemic choice is to pull rank or double down on epistemic dialogue, I argue in this chapter that we ought to double down. My argument asks that we stay open to learning new things. This request means we must accept that we will sometimes learn the wrong things, but within this acceptance is hope, not resignation. For just as we know we will sometimes get things wrong, we also retain the ability to learn new things, to be surprised, to have our epistemology remain nimble in the face of unexpected events or information. Put differently, my argument asks not only for openness but also for inclusion. We must remain open to learning new things so that we can be inclusive of a wide range of perspectives, so we can find truth even in unlikely places.

This general argument mirrors the more specific one I've been making with respect to patient-centered measures: these instruments should prioritize patient involvement through epistemic dialogue, and they should be inclusive of a range of respondent answers through the ongoing coordination of instruments and constructs.

Seen in this light, as an example of a more general point about learning and inclusion, patient-centered measures represent an opportunity to stand as a benchmark of epistemic and ethical excellence, that is, to really become vehicles, not only for patient-centered care, but also for humility and collaboration. While it is true that patient-centered measurement doesn't eliminate the possibility of pharmaceutical industry's influence, it does offer a response. In fact, it offers two. Epistemic dialogue provides an opportunity to bring to light the assumptions and values that industry brings to measurement; it provides an opportunity for critical engagement that goes beyond a narrow evaluation of scientific rigor. On the other hand, ongoing coordination give us second, third, fourth—10 billionth—chances to do better, be better, to see more clearly what is at stake in the interplay between part and whole, our past and our future.

Conclusion

When I was in high school our library purchased a bunch of stereograms, two-dimensional images that use the difference in perspective between your left and right eye to create the illusion of a three-dimensional image. We crowded around them to see what we could see. Appreciating the three-dimensional image in a stereogram takes practice, and at first all I saw was the flat image. Eventually, I could hold the three-dimensional image for a few seconds before it collapsed back down. Over time I got better at it and could hold the image for longer periods, but eventually it too would collapse back into a two-dimensional image, and there I was, once again, straining to see a dinosaur leap from the page. Writing *Patient-Centered Measurement* has sometimes felt like looking into a stereogram. My vision flips between different points of view: my claims seem risky and unorthodox and then, suddenly, conventional and obvious.

Sometimes I see as unconventional my view that patient-centered measures are instruments with revolutionary power to sensitize our evidence base to human needs and interests and make patient care more personal, perhaps even roll back the 18th-century "disappearance" of patient voices that Nicolas Jewson (1976) and Mary Fissell (1991) discuss in their work.[1] Other times, I think these ideas are nothing more than the long-held motivations for national health policies in countries like the United States, United Kingdom, and Denmark. Sometimes I see as unorthodox my epistemic theory of patient-centered measures, which, instead of theorizing about patient-centered constructs, governs patients' and other contributions to measure development. Sometimes I think prioritizing patients with epistemic dialogue and creating more inclusive measures with ongoing coordination is innovative. Other times I see these ideas as simply dressing up existing initiatives (e.g., FDA, Program PRO) or just emphasizing with co-ordination what we've long been told about validity: it's an ongoing process (e.g., Rothrock et al. 2011). Even my hermeneutic approach, which I am very fond of, has some days felt like a mash-up of the work from my favorite historians of science.

Patient-Centered Measurement. Leah M. McClimans, Oxford University Press. © Oxford University Press 2024.
DOI: 10.1093/oso/9780197572078.003.0008

At times like these, I take comfort from authors as diverse as Mark Twain and Audrey Lorde (1984), who tell us that new ideas are nonexistent and impossible. Twain's biographer Albert Bigelow Paine (1912, 1341) quotes Twain as saying,

> There is no such thing as a new idea. It is impossible. We simply take a lot of old ideas and put them into a sort of mental kaleidoscope. We give them a turn and they make new and curious combinations indefinitely; but they are the same old pieces of colored glass that have been in use through all the ages.

I love Twain's image of the mental kaleidoscope (kaleidoscopes: much easier than stereograms). Yet kaleidoscopes can be tricky. Turn it too much and the ideas you get will be incomprehensible (too far from what we know), turn it too little and they will be uninteresting (too familiar). Writing compelling philosophy is, I think, largely a matter of walking an uncharted line down the middle: shake up those old ideas, but not too much, not too little. So, on my good days, I think the flipping vision between a two- and three-dimensional *Patient-Centered Measurement* stereogram has satisfied the goals with which I began. Today is a good day.

In this book, I wanted to make questionnaires interesting, to show how asking questions as a means of measurement is a fascinating, multifaceted subject that can take us to all kinds of wonderful and perhaps unexpected places. Questions are fascinating, but we tend to ignore them—in philosophy, health science, *life*—in favor of answers. If ever there is an opportunity to reverse this course, it has to be with *question*naires. Taking questions seriously as a conceptual tool is like finding a missing piece to a puzzle: it clarifies the significance of our work. It helps us to see, for instance, what is at stake when we standardize questions. Part of preparing to take questions more seriously meant excavating patient-centered measures away from some of our entrenched disciplinary assumptions about them. Chapters 1 and 2 are my attempt to break up those assumptions. Chapters 3 and 4, then, allow me to recontextualize these measures in different terms: in terms of questions and in terms of ethics. Patient-centered measures have much ethical promise, but they are also ethically perilous. Yet ethics is not the "lingua franca" of patient-centered measures. It should be more so. I wanted a chapter that cast these measures in ethical language from beginning to end, both to illustrate the ethical dimensions involved and to perhaps seduce those who work with these measures to speak in these terms. While Chapters 3 and 4 aim to recontextualize patient-centered measures, Chapters 5 and 6 take these reconstituted instruments and see how they fare when I plant them back in the fields of everyday concerns.

Although my overarching aim was to make questionnaires interesting, I also wanted to make my approach *believable*. So these chapters contain a number of concrete examples of patient-centered measurement policies, guidelines, and empirical studies from the health science literature. These examples are my tethers to familiar (or at least peer-previewed) ideas. If my journey into ethics and questions brings patient-centered measures into new relationships, then these examples aim to illustrate the legitimacy of these relationships. I'm sure that, for some, these examples go too far, and for others, they don't go far enough. Such is the difficulty of interdisciplinary research. But I do want to address one question some of these examples raise, the answer to which has so far been vague.

In Chapters 4–6, I suggest the use of appraisal metrics to aid in ongoing coordination of patient-centered measures. I offer some possibilities for how this might work. We might use appraisal information to adjust our interpretation of measurement outcomes for some subpopulation. This use could perhaps be similar to the way uncertainty budgets work with cesium fountains. Or, in light of appraisal outcomes, we might alter patient-centered measures themselves to better reflect respondent understandings, perhaps redefining the construct of interest—splitting it into two constructs or reconceptualizing it altogether. My suggestions here are perhaps instances where my empirical examples don't go far enough for some readers. How precisely would my suggestion work? What would be the methodology involved? The short answer to these questions: I don't know.

On the one hand, response shift research, and the appraisal model in particular, is still very much part of a young and evolving field. Not all of the interesting questions have been answered or even explored, especially applications of appraisal. Much of the literature to date has focused on legitimating response shift as an important phenomenon when measuring change (e.g., Swartz et al. 2011), developing methods to detect it (e.g., Sébille et al. 2021), and theorizing and modeling it (e.g., Rapkin and Schwartz 2004; Vanier et al. 2021). How appraisal might aid, precisely, in the ongoing coordination of patient-centered measures is a particularly interesting suggestion exactly because we don't yet have a settled answer.

On the other hand, when I offer up appraisal metrics as a plausible suggestion to ground ongoing coordination, this offering isn't entirely unprecedented. In the response shift literature the use of appraisal measures has often focused on improving clinical care with individual patients. But uses similar to those I suggest in the context of ongoing coordination have also been made. Schwartz and colleagues (2007) have suggested that appraisal outcomes could lead to the modification of items, or the development of protocols or algorithms to assess response shift. The use of these findings could then aid in the interpretation or "adjustment" of scores. My hope is that my suggestion to use appraisal metrics to aid ongoing coordination might spur further interest in this application.

Finally, if there is one aspect of this book that I always think is unorthodox and risky, it's the application of Gadamer's hermeneutics to analytic philosophy of measurement. If you've stuck with me this far, I want to thank you. From the first time I read van Fraassen's (2008) explanation of coordination as having the structure of a hermeneutic circle I knew I was going to have to write a book about it. Few philosophers of science want to talk about Gadamer, let alone read about him. But if patient-centered measures need an ethical vocabulary, then I think philosophers of science would have richer conceptual resources if they opened up to new historical sources. Gadamer has always been a fellow traveler, and I hope I have convinced some of you of the depth of his insights while also writing, more or less, in plain English.

Patient-centered measures are important, and *Patient-Centered Measurement* aims to bring our philosophy of these measures into the 21st century. This is a century where patients' points of view matter, not just rhetorically but really. In policy. In regulation. In research. In the clinic. When I first encountered these measures (in a small scanning room at the Royal College of Surgeons in London), I had a hunch that something different was at stake, something that big numbers couldn't—and yes, shouldn't—wash out. I had a hunch that these measures variously referred to as quality of life measures and patient-reported outcomes measures were distinct from other measures in the human sciences because they embodied an ethical orientation that took patient perspectives seriously. *Patient-Centered Measurement* is the culmination of my hunch. If other measures have reason to take first-person perspectives seriously, if the epistemic theory of patient-centered measurement has reason to travel to other measures to humanize and diversify, then—all the better! Fertility is a virtue of philosophy, as it is of science.

Notes

The Puzzle

1. Patient-centered measures are also used increasingly in the clinical arena, where they can be implemented to improve the individualization of patient care and patient-clinician communication.

Chapter 1

1. Shout out to Eran Tal and Becca Johnson for making me aware of this literature.
2. Thank you to Suman Seth for giving me with this reference.
3. Although some researchers have tried to improve interpretability by improving measurement theory or by other statistical means (e.g., Jaescheke et al. 1989), I argue toward the end of this chapter and elsewhere (McClimans 2011) that these attempts have only been marginally successful.
4. Personal correspondence.
5. Thank you to Suman Seth for this helpful transition.
6. Indeed, some have argued that CTT is unfalsifiable (Borsboom 2005; Hobart et al. 2007). Borsboom (2005) calls CTT a "tautology."
7. In this discussion I leave to one side questions of structural validity, i.e., the degree to which a scale's items are related to one another. To be sure, Cronbach and Meehl (1955, 288) recognize that structural validity can be a source of evidence for construct validity. Depending on the theory of the construct of interest, different levels of item correlation can support the inference that an instrument measures the construct intended. For a philosophical account of structural validity see Alexandrova 2017, 139–40.
8. There is debate over whether the Rasch model can in fact be taken as a form of additive conjoint measurement. See, for instance, Borsboom and Mellenbergh 2004; Borsboom and Scholten 2008; Michell 2000.
9. We should not be misled by the fact that this approach is officially discredited. As I discussed in the context of CTT, it is common for discussions of validity to demand theoretical justification, while sanctioned practical applications carry on without it.
10. Thank you to John Browne for driving this point home—usually while driving us home.

Chapter 2

1. To be clear, I am not suggesting that patient-centered measures are independent from questions about well-being, i.e., how well life is going for a population of people. On the contrary, patient-centered measures are, in a general sense, quite obviously concerned with how life is going for patients. But I do not think that much follows, theoretically, from this acknowledgment.
2. For a philosophical discussion of this issue see McClimans 2010b, 2011.
3. Elizabeth Barnes (2016) does an excellent job of summarizing this literature.
4. For a discussion of how, in practice, the capability approach applied to quality of life and PROMs tends to conflate functionings with disability and chronic illness, see McClimans 2010a.

Chapter 3

1. In philosophy "prudential" is a type of value that contrasts with moral values or aesthetic values. Prudential value refers to what is good for a person. It is often identified with well-being. Prudential theories are theories of well-being, theories like objective list theory or hedonism.
2. It may be that Alexandrova's view on patient participation is evolving. In a recent article she argues for the co-production of thick concepts, such as well-being, for the purpose of measurement (see Alexandrova and Fabian 2022).
3. Qualitative research isn't just important for understanding quality of life with epilepsy, see Snow, Humphrey and Sandall (2013) for an example that illustrates its use for Diabetes.
4. In fact, we don't need to imagine these scenarios. In a 2010 cross-sectional study of 9,159 Egyptian women, Dalal et al. found that 82% favored the continuation of female circumcision. In her MA thesis for the University of Manitoba, Kendra Monk (2014) interviewed six couples from Winnipeg, and Brown and Brown's 1987 study emphasizes social concerns as reasons for male circumcision (see also Mazor 2013).

Chapter 4

1. There are, of course, other dimensions to inclusivity that I do not address in this chapter: weighting item scores in ways that do not reflect respondent priorities, the burden of responding to patient-centered measures, and so on. Thanks to Eran Tal for this point.
2. This is not to say there haven't been attempts to address theoretical issues of response shift; see, for instance, Rapkin and Schwartz 2004, 2019; Vanier et al. 2021.

3. In draft guidance the Food and Drug Administration (FDA) (2022) has defined fit for purpose differently. They define fit-for-purpose as "the level of validation associated with a medical product development tool is sufficient to support its context of use." On this definition fit-for-purpose is determined by two considerations: 1) concept of interest and context of use are clearly described and 2) there is sufficient evidence to support the rationale for the prosed interpretation and use of the measure.

4. I am assuming a reflective measurement model; this is the common assumption within psychological measurement.

5. To be sure, questionnaires are never wholly successful in representing the constructs or latent traits they aim to measure. As with all measures, patient-centered measures are subject to error. Nevertheless, the aim is to create ever more accurate instruments.

6. "Gender specific biological conditions" is Hagquist's phrase, not mine.

7. As Hagquist (2019) explains, resolving an item in group comparisons has the same effect as removing the item. The stomachache item has different gender specific location and/or slope values; the group estimates are no longer invariant.

8. To be sure, disorders such as psychosomatic disorder have been characterized by their symptoms in publications like the International Classification of Diseases-11 (World Health Organization 2022) and the Diagnostic and Statistical Manual of Mental Disorders-5 (American Psychiatric Association 2013). But at best these classifications are definitions used for diagnosis; they are not robust conceptualizations that utilize theoretical language to explore these disorders. Such a conceptualization would use observable and unobservable variables to create hypotheses. They might also make explicit the values—both epistemic and non-epistemic—that function to characterize the disorder.

9. To be sure locating a person or population within a topic of interest is, in a manner of speaking, to learn something new. Standardized questions are not merely rhetorical: we ask them in order to learn something about the people answering them. But standardized questions are not used to learn something new about the topic of the question.

10. Van Fraassen (1980), like Rapkin and Schwartz, draws our attention to the contextual features of interrogatives to illuminate what question is being expressed (McClimans 2011). Where van Fraassen discusses contrast classes, Rapkin and Schwartz discuss standards of comparison; where van Fraassen speaks of relevance relations, Rapkin and Schwartz refer to frames of reference and sampling of experiences. Moreover, just as van Fraassen resisted limiting those relevance relations that can count as scientific (much to the dismay of some philosophers of science; see Kitcher and Salmon 1987), Rapkin and Schwartz have resisted mechanical objectivity. Together they acknowledge that interpretation is important to evaluating answers to questions.

11. Although it is true that this point has not received as much attention in philosophy of measurement as, I think, it deserves, it is a point that has currency elsewhere. In *Science in Action* (1987, 250–52) Bruno Latour argues that the stability of time is due to the constant extension of a network of linkages between the clocks we use to tell

time through to primary and secondary clocks through to abstract physical concepts. Special thanks to Eran Tal for connecting this point to my own.

Chapter 5

1. Hausman (2015, 47) disagrees.
2. Some argue that for the vast majority of emergency department patients, smaller, low-volume hospitals do not provide worse care (Vaughan and Browne 2022).
3. Alexandrova, similar to Hausman, is predominately interested in interpersonal heterogeneity and response shift focuses on intrapersonal heterogeneity. Nonetheless, the response shift literature provide insights into interpersonal heterogeneity over time. Moreover, whether intra- or interpersonal, heterogeneity poses measurement questions that ought to be considered.
4. I do not endorse wholesale this three-way distinction among performance, perception, and evaluative measures. To be sure, as I discussed in the previous chapter, there are cases when, for practical purposes, e.g., pedagogy, a topic of interest and the questions that refer to it are standardized. That is, the topic is not open to reinterpretation; answers to questions are right or wrong based on a fixed interpretation. Consequently, for some purposes and within some time frames, measures function as Rapkin and Schwartz suggest "performance" or "perception" measures do in that the relationship between the construct and questions remains the same over time and among respondents. But I don't think these constructs are *forever* closed to reinterpretation. Indeed, the history of science suggests otherwise. I do think there are interesting questions about who is recognized as a relevant contributor and is thus able to effect this kind of interpretive change (who is expert?). In the context of patient-centered measures, which I focus in this book, the "who" are patients, people with disabilities, and other ill persons in conjunction with clinicians and other health researchers.
5. Small effect sizes can matter in understanding the impact of treatment or psychological factor. Moreover, the cumulative effect of small effects can lead to medium effects that pass criteria for clinical significance (Schwartz, personal correspondence, 2022).
6. Big thank you to Mark Fabian, who suggested this conceptualization to me, and the "Measuring the Human: New Developments in the Epistemology of Measurement in the Human Sciences" conference at the University of Cambridge, Department of History and Philosophy of Science, July 2023, that brought us together in the nick of time.
7. Assuming we don't already activate appraisal processes during the internal assessment of the construct or latent trait.

Chapter 6

1. To be sure, this statistic can be manipulated by increasing the sample size. The greater the sample size the smaller the standard error around the item estimates and the less likely for overlap to occur.
2. The ADAS-cog includes both respondent questions and observer questions.
3. This isn't to say there hasn't been bad science funded by industry or science with the aim of distorting a reality that is damaging to industry (see Oreskes and Conway 2010; Elliot 2018).
4. Indeed, in the conference Holman recounts above, industry representatives were seeking guidelines for how to present to the FDA evidence of efficacy.

Conclusion

1. Thank you Suman!

References

Abma, Inger L., Maroeska Rovers, and Philip J. van der Wees. 2016. "Appraising Convergent Validity of Patient-Reported Outcome Measures in Systematic Reviews: Constructing Hypotheses and Interpreting Outcomes." *BMC Research Notes* 9: 2–5.

Acquadro, Catherine, Rick Berzon, Dominique Dubois, Nancy Klein Leidy, Patrick Marquis, Dennis Revicki, Margaret Rothman, and PRO Harmonization Group. 2003. "Incorporating the Patient's Perspective into Drug Development and Communication: An Ad Hoc Task Force Report of the Patient-Reported Outcomes (PRO) Harmonizations Group Meeting at the Food and Drug Administration, February 16, 2001." *Value in Health* 6 (5): 522–31.

Alcoff, Linda Martín. 2007. "Epistemologies of Ignorance: Three Types." In *Race and Epistemologies of Ignorance*, edited by Shannon Sullivan and Nancy Tuana, 39–58. New York: SUNY Press.

Alder, Ken. 2003. *The Measure of All Things: The Seven-Year Odyssey and Hidden Error That Transformed the World*. Chicago: Free Press.

Alexandrova, Anna. 2017. *A Philosophy for the Science of Well-Being*. Oxford: Oxford University Press.

Alexandrova, Anna and Mark Fabian. 2022. "Democratising Measurement: Or Why Thick Concepts Call for Coproduction." *European Journal for Philosophy of Science* 12 (7).

Alexandrova, Anna and Daniel M. Haybron. 2016. "Is Construct Validation Valid?" *Philosophy of Science* 83 (5): 1098–109.

American Educational Research Association, American Psychological Association, and National Council on Measurement in Education. 2014. *Standards for Education and Psychological Testing*. Washington, DC: American Educational Research Association.

American Psychiatric Association. 2013. *Diagnostic and Statistical Manual of Mental Disorders*. 5th ed. Arlington, VA: American Psychiatric Association.

Angner, Erik. 2011. "The Evolution of Eupathics: The Historical Roots of Subjective Measures of Wellbeing." *International Journal of Wellbeing* 1 (1): 4–41.

Apgar, Virginia. 1953. "A Proposal for a New Method of Evaluation of the Newborn Infant." *Current Research in Anesthesia and Analgesia* 32 (4): 260–67.

Aaronson, Neil, Sam Ahmedzai, Bengt Bergman, Monika Bullinger, Ann Cull, Nicole Duez, Antonio Filiberti, Henning Flechtner, and Stewart Fleishman. 1993. "The European Organization for Research and Treatment of Cancer QLQ-C30: A Quality-of-Life Instrument for Use in International Clinical Trials in Oncology." *Journal of the National Cancer Institute* 85 (5): 365–76.

Barclay-Goddard, Ruth, Joshua D. Epstein, and Nancy E. Mayo. 2009. "Response Shift: A Brief Overview and Proposed Research Priorities." *Quality of Life Research* 18 (3): 335–46.

Barnes, Elizabeth. 2016. *The Minority Body: A Theory of Disability*. Oxford: Oxford University Press.

Basso, Alessandra. 2017. "The Appeal to Robustness in Measurement Practice." *Studies in the History and Philosophy of Science* 65–66: 57–66.

Beckman, Howard B. and Richard M. Frankel. 1984. "The Effect of Physician Behavior on the Collection of Data." *Annals of Internal Medicine* 101 (5): 692–96.

Bernstein, Richard J. 1982. "What Is the Difference That Makes a Difference? Gadamer, Habermas and Rorty." *PSA: Proceedings of the Biennial Meeting of the Philosophy of Science Association* 1982 (2): 331–59.

Besley, John C., Aaron M. McCright, Nagwan R. Zahry, Kevin C. Elliott, Norbert E. Kaminski, and Joseph D. Martin. 2017. "Perceived Conflict of Interest in Health Science Partnerships." *PLoS One* 12 (4): e0175643.

Biddle, Justin. 2013. "Institutionalizing Dissent: A Proposal for an Adversarial System of Pharmaceutical Research." *Kennedy Institute of Ethics Journal* 23 (4): 325–53.

Biddle, Justin. 2016. "Inductive Risk, Epistemic Risk and Overdiagnosis of Disease." *Perspectives on Science* 24 (2): 192–205.

Black, Nick. 2013. "Patient Reported Outcome Measures Could Transform Healthcare." *British Medical Journal* 346: f167.

Bohlig, Michael, William Fisher, Geoff Masters, and Trevor Bond. 1998. "Content Validity, Construct Validity and Misfitting Items." *Rasch Measurement Transactions* 12: 607.

Borsboom, Denny. 2005. *Measuring the Mind*. Cambridge: Cambridge University Press.

Borsboom, Denny. 2006. "Attack of the Psychometricians." *Psychometrika* 71: 425–40.

Borsboom, Denny and Gideon J. Mellenbergh. 2004. "Why Psychometrics Is Not Pathological: A Comment on Michell." *Theory & Psychology* 14: 105–20.

Borsboom, Denny and Annemarie Zand Scholten. 2008. "The Rasch Model and Conjoint Measurement Theory from the Perspective of Psychometrics." *Theory & Psychology* 18 (1): 111–17.

Boyer, Laurent, Karin Baumstarck, Eric Guedj, and Pascal Auquier. 2014. "What's Wrong with Quality-of-Life Measures? A Philosophical Reflection and Insights from Neuroimaging." *Expert Review of Pharmacoeconomics & Outcomes Research* 14: 767–69.

Bradburn, Norman, Nancy Cartwright, and Jonathan Fuller. 2017. "A Theory of Measurement." In *Measurement in Medicine: Philosophical Essays on Assessment and Evaluation*, edited by Leah McClimans, 73–88. London: Rowman & Littlefield.

Breslau, Joshua, Kristin Javaras, Deborah Blacker, and Jane Murphy. 2008. "Differential Item Functioning between Ethnic Groups in the Epidemiological Assessment of Depression." *Journal of Nervous and Mental Disease* 196 (4): 297–306.

Brock, Dan. 1993. "Quality of Life Measures in Health Care and Medical Ethics." In *The Quality of Life*, edited by Martha Nussbaum and Amartya Sen, 95–132. Oxford: Clarendon Press.

Brodie, Martin J. and Jacqueline A. French. 2000. "Management of Epilepsy in Adolescents and Adults." *The Lancet* 356: 323–29.

Brogden, Hubert E. 1977. "The Rasch Model, the Law of Comparative Judgment, and Additive Conjoint Measurement." *Psychometrika* 42: 631–35.

Brow, John P., Hannah M. McGee, and Ciaran A. O'Boyle. 1997. "Conceptual Approaches to the Assessment of Quality of Life." *Psychology & Health* 12 (6): 737–51.

Brown, Mark S. and Cheryl A. Brown. 1987. "Circumcision Decision: Prominence of Social Concerns." *Pediatrics* 80 (2): 215–19.

Browne John Patrick, Cano Stefan C., and Smith Sarah. 2017. "Using Patient-Reported Outcome Measures to Improve Healthcare: Time for a New Approach." *Medical Care* 55 (10): 901–04.

Bueter, Anke and Saana Jukola. 2020. "Sex, Drugs, and How to Deal with Criticism: The Case of Flibanserin." In *Uncertainty in Pharmacology, Epistemology, Methods and Decisions*, edited by Adam LaCaze and Barbara Osimani, 451–69. Cham, Switzerland: Springer Nature.

Buist, Michael. 2014. "Instead of Writing Policy and Procedure We in the NHS Should Learn to Listen." *The Guardian*, December 12, 2014. https://www.theguardian.com/hea lthcare-network/views-from-the-nhs-frontline/2014/dec/15/nhs-staff-learn-listen.

BIPM. 2019. Le Système international d'unités/The International System of Unites ("The SI Brochure") (updated 2022). Bureau international des poids et mesures, 9th ed. http://www.bipm.org/en/si/si_brochure/.

Campbell, Norman Robert. 1920. *Physics: The Elements*. Cambridge: Cambridge University Press.

Cano, Stefan J. and Jeremy C. Hobart. 2011. "The Problem with Health Measurement." *Patient Preference and Adherence* 5: 279–90.

Cano, Stefan J., Holly B. Posner, Margaret L. Moline, Stephen W. Hurt, Jina Swartz, Tim Hsu, and Jeremey C. Hobart. 2010. "The ADAS-cog in Alzheimer's Disease Clinical Trials: Psychometric Evaluation of the Sum and Its Parts." *Journal of Neurology, Neurosurgery, and Psychiatry* 81 (12): 1363–68.

Carr, Allison J. and Irene J. Higginson. 2001. "Are Quality of Life Measures Patient Centred?" *British Medical Journal* 322: 1357–60.

Cartwright, Nancy. 2020. "Middle-Range Theory: Without It What Could Anyone Do?" *Theoria* 35 (3): 269–323.

Cella, David, David T. Eton, Jin-Shei Lai, Amy Peterman, and Douglas E. Merkel. 2002. "Combining Anchor and Distribution-Based Methods to Derive Minimal Clinically Important Differences on the Functional Assessment of Cancer Therapy (FACT) Anemia and Fatigue Scales." *Journal of Pain and Symptom Measurement* 24 (6): 547–61.

Chang, Hasok. 2004. *Inventing Temperature: Measurement and Scientific Progress*. Oxford: Oxford University Press.

Chong, Lauren, Nathan Jamieson, Deepak Gill, Davinder Singh-Grewal, Jonathan Craig, Angela Ju, Camilla S. Hanson, and Allison Tong. 2016. "Children's Experiences of Epilepsy: A Systematic Review of Qualitative Studies." *Pediatrics* 138 (3): e20160658.

Cleanthous, Sophie, Skye Pamela Barbic, Sarah Smith, and Antonie Regnault. 2019. "Psychometric Performance of the PROMIS® Depression Item Bank: A Comparison of the 28- and 51-Item Versions Using Rasch Measurement Theory." *Journal of Patient-Reported Outcomes* 3 (1): 47.

Code, Lorraine. 2003. "Introduction: Why Feminists Do Not Read Gadamer." In *Feminist Interpretations of Hans-Georg Gadamer*, edited by Lorraine Code, 1–36. University Park: Pennsylvania State University Press.

Craig, Edward. 1990. *Knowledge and the State of Nature: An Essa in Conceptual Synthesis*. Oxford: Clarendon Press.

Critical Path Institute. n.d. "About." Accessed September 2022. https://c-path.org/about/.

Crocker, Thomas F., Jamie K. Smith, and Suzanne M. Skevington. 2015. "Family and Professionals Underestimate Quality of Life across Diverse Cultures and Health Conditions: Systematic Review." *Journal of Clinical Epidemiology* 68: 584–95.

Cronbach, Lee J. and Paul E. Meehl. 1955. "Construct Validity in Psychological Tests." *Psychological Bulletin* 52: 281–302.

Dalal, Koustuv, Stephen Lawoko, and Bjarne Jansson. 2010. "Women's Attitudes towards Discontinuation of Female Genital Mutilation in Egypt." *Injury and Violence* 2 (1): 41–47.

Daniels, Norman. 1981. "Health-Care Needs and Distributive Justice." *Philosophy & Public Affairs* 10 (2): 146–79.

Danto, Arthur C. 1965. *Analytical Philosophy of History.* Cambridge: Cambridge University Press.

Darzi, Lord. 2008. "Summary Letter." In *High Quality Care for All: NHS Next Stage Review, Final Report*, 7–15. London: The Stationary Office.

Daston, Lorraine and Peter Galison. 2007. *Objectivity.* New York: Zone Books.

de Vet, Henrica C. W., Caroline B. Terwee, Libwine B. Mokkink, and Dirk L. Knol. 2011. *Measurement in Medicine: A Practical Guide.* Cambridge: Cambridge University Press.

Devlin, Nancy and John Appleby. 2010. *Getting the Most out of PROMs: Putting Health Outcomes at the Heart of NHS Decision-Making.* London: King's Fund.

Devlin, Nancy and Richard Brooks. 2017. "The EQ-5D and the EuroQol Group: Past, Present and Future." *Applied Health Economics and Health Policy* 15 (2): 127–37.

Diener, Ed. 1984. "Subjective Well-Being." *Psychological Bulletin* 95 (3): 542–75.

Diener, Ed and Richard Lucas. 1999. "Personality and Subjective Well-Being." In *Well-Being: The Foundations of Hedonic Psychology*, edited by Daniel E. Kahneman, Ed Diener, and Norbert Schwarz, 213–29. New York: Russell Sage.

Diener, Ed, Eunkook M. Suh, Richard E. Lucas, and Heidi L. Smith. 1999. "Subjective Well-Being: Three Decades of Progress." *Psychological Bulletin* 125 (2): 276–302.

Donabedian, Avedis. 2005. "Evaluating the Quality of Medical Care." *Milbank Quarterly* 83 (4): 691–729.

Donovan, Jenny, Stephen Frankel, and John Eyles. 1993. "Assessing the Need for Health Status Measures." *Journal of Epidemiology and Community Health* 47 (2): 158–62.

Douglas, Heather. 2004. "The Irreducible Complexity of Objectivity." *Synthese* 138 (3): 453–73.

Douglas, Heather. 2009. *Science, Policy and the Value-Free Ideal.* Pittsburgh: University of Pittsburgh Press.

Douglas, Jeffrey, Louis Roussos, and William Stout. 1996. "Item Bundle DIF Hypothesis Testing: Identifying Suspect Bundles and Assessing Their Differential Functioning." *Journal of Educational Measurement* 33 (4): 465–84.

Durez, Patrick, Virginie Fraselle, Frédéric Houssiau, Jean-Louis Thonnard, Henri Nielens, and Massimo Penta. 2007. "Validation of the ABILHAND Questionnaire as a Measure of Manual Ability in Patients with Rheumatoid Arthritis." *Annals of the Rheumatic Diseases* 66 (8): 1098–105.

Earp, Brian D. 2017. "Does Female Genital Mutilation Have Health Benefits? The Problem with Medicalizing Morality." *Journal of Medical Ethics* blog, August 15. https://blogs. bmj.com/medical-ethics/2017/08/15/does-female-genital-mutilation-have-health-benefits-the-problem-with-medicalizing-morality/.

Edwards, Michael C., Ashley Slagle, Jonathan D. Rubright, and R. J. Wirth. 2018. "Fit for Purpose and Modern Validity Theory in Clinical Outcomes Assessment." *Quality of Life Research* 27: 1711–20.

Efstathiou, Sophia. 2012. "How Ordinary Race Concepts Get to Be Usable in Biomedical Science: An Account of Founded Race Concepts." *Philosophy of Science* 79 (5): 701–13.

Efstathiou, Sophia. 2016. "Is It Possible to Give Scientific Solutions to Grand Challenges? On the Idea of Grand Challenges for Life Science Research." *Studies in History and Philosophy of Science Part C: Studies in History and Philosophy of Biological and Biomedical Sciences* 56: 48–61.

Egholm, Cecilie Lindström, Sanne Jensen, Annette Wandel, and Mogens Hørder. 2023. "The Implementation of the 2017 National Policy on Patient-Reported Outcomes in Denmark: An Overview of Developments after Six Years." *Health Policy* 130: 104755.

Elliot, Kevin. 2018. "Addressing Industry-Funded Research with Criteria for Objectivity." *Philosophy of Science* 85 (5): 857–68.

Fabian, Mark. 2022. "Scale Norming Undermines the Use of Life Satisfaction Scale Data for Welfare Analysis." *Journal of Happiness Studies* 23: 1509–41.

Faden, Ruth R. and Tom L. Beauchamp. 1986. *A History and Theory of Informed Consent.* Oxford: Oxford University Press.

Fadiman, Anne. 1997. *The Spirit Catches You and You Fall Down: A Hmong Child, Her American Doctors, and the Collision of Two Cultures.* New York: Farrar, Straus, and Giroux.

Fairclough, Diane L. 2017. "Challenges of Interpreting Patient Reported Outcomes from Clinical Trials." *Annals of Translational Medicine* 5 (20): 408.

Fayed, Nora, Aileen M. Davis, David L. Streiner, Peter L. Rosenbaum, Charles E. Cunningham, Lucyna M. Lach, Michael H. Boyle, Gabriel M. Ronen, and QUALITÉ Study Group. 2015. "Children's Perspective of Quality of Life in Epilepsy." *Neurology* 84 (18): 1830–37.

Fayers, Peter and Andrew Bottomley on behalf of the EORTC Quality of Life Group and the Quality of Life Unit. 2002. "Quality of Life Research within the EORTC—EORTC QLQ-C30." *European Journal of Cancer* 38 (4): 125–33.

Fayers, Peter M. and David Machin. 2000. *Quality of Life: Assessment, Analysis and Interpretation.* Hoboken, NJ: John Wiley & Sons.

Fayers, Peter M. and David Machin. 2007. *Quality of Life, the Assessment, Analysis and Interpretation of Patient-Reported Outcomes.* 2nd ed. Chichester: Wiley Press.

Fenández Pinto, Manuela. 2014. "Philosophy of Science for Globalized Privatization: Uncovering Some Limitations of Critical Contextual Empiricism." *Studies in History and Philosophy of Science Part A* 47: 10–17.

Finnis, John. 2011. *Natural Law and Natural Rights.* 2nd ed. Oxford: Clarendon Press.

Fissell, Mary. 1991. "The Disappearance of Patient's Narrative and the Invention of Hospital Medicine." In *British Medicine in the Age of Reform*, edited by Roger French and Andrew Wear, 92–109. London: Routledge.

Food and Drug Administration (FDA). 2009. "Guidance for Industry on Patient-Reported Outcomes Measures: Use in Medicinal Product Development to Support Labeling Claims." *Federal Register* 74: 1–43.

Food and Drug Administration (FDA). 2017. "Plan for Issuance of Patient-Focused Drug Development Guidance." https://www.fda.gov/downloads/forindustry/userfees/pres criptiondruguserfee/ucm563618.pdf.

Food and Drug Administration (FDA). 2020. "Assessing User Fees under the Prescription Drug User Fee Amendments of 2017: Guidance for Industry." https://www.fda.gov/ media/108233/download.

Food and Drug Administration (FDA). 2020. "Learn about FDA Patient Engagement." Last modified March 16, 2020. https://www.fda.gov/patients/learn-more-about-pati ent-engagement.

Food and Drug Administration (FDA). 2022. "FDA-Led Patient-Focused Drug Development (PFDD) Public Meetings." Last modified July 18, 2022. https://www.fda.gov/industry/prescription-drug-user-fee-amendments/fda-led-patient-focused-drug-development-pfdd-public-meetings.

Food and Drug Administration (FDA). 2022c. "Drug Development Tool (DDT) Qualification Programs." Last modified July 7, 2022. https://www.fda.gov/drugs/development-approval-process-drugs/drug-development-tool-ddt-qualification-programs.

Food and Drug Administration (FDA). 2022d. "Patient-Focused Drug Development: Selecting, Developing, or Modifying Fit-for-Purpose Clinical Outcome Assessments. Guidance of Industry, Food and Drug Administration Staff, and Other Stakeholders Draft Guidance." Last modified June 30, 2022. https://www.fda.gov/regulatory-information/search-fda-guidance-documents/patient-focused-drug-development-selecting-developing-or-modifying-fit-purpose-clinical-outcome.

Food and Drug Administration (FDA). 2023. "FDA Patient Focused Drug Development Guidance Series for Enhancing the Incorporation of the Patient's Voice in Medical Product Development and Regulatory Decision Making." Last modified April 6, 2023. https://www.fda.gov/drugs/development-approval-process-drugs/fda-patient-focused-drug-development-guidance-series-enhancing-incorporation-patients-voice-medical.

Food and Drug Administration (FDA). n.d. "Advisory Committees." Accessed October 2022. https://www.fda.gov/advisory-committees.

Foucault, Michel. 1963/1973. Birth of the Clinic. Translated by Alan Sheridan. New York: Pantheon Books.

Foucault, Michel. 1975/1977. Discipline and Punish: The Birth of the Prison. Translated by Alan Sheridan. New York: Pantheon Books.

Frank, Arthur. 2003. The Wounded Storyteller Body, Illness, and Ethics. 2nd ed. Chicago: University of Chicago Press.

Fricker, Miranda. 2007. Epistemic Injustice Power and the Ethics of Knowing. Oxford: Oxford University Press.

Gadamer, Hans-Georg. 2004. Truth and Method. Translated by Joel Weinsheimer and Donald G. Marshall. New York: Continuum Press.

Galison, Peter. 1999. "Trading Zone: Coordinating Action and Belief." In The Science Studies Reader, edited by Mario Biagioli, 137–60. New York: Routledge.

Gellad, Walid, F, Kathryn E. Flynn, and Caleb Alexander. 2015. "Evaluation of Flibanserin Science and Advocacy at the FDA." Journal of the American Medical Association 314 (9): 869–70.

George, Theodore. 2021. "Hermeneutics." In The Stanford Encyclopedia of Philosophy, edited by Edward N. Zalta. https://plato.stanford.edu/archives/win2021/entries/hermeneutics/.

Goldenberg, Maya. 2016. "Public Misunderstanding of Science? Reframing the Problem of Vaccine Hesitancy." Perspectives on Science 24 (5): 552–81.

Goldenberg, Maya. 2021. Vaccine Hesitancy: Public Trust, Expertise, and the War on Science. Pittsburgh: University of Pittsburgh Press.

Goldenberg, Paul. 2020. "Classroom Stories: Correct Answer, Wrong Question." Elementary Math at EDC (blog). Educational Development Center. https://elementarymath.edc.org/resources/correct-answer-wrong-question-theory-of-mind-in-a-mathematics-class/.

Griffin, James. 1986. *Well-Being: Its Meaning, Measurement, and Moral Importance.* Oxford: Clarendon Press.

Grondin, Jean. 1997. *Introduction to Philosophical Hermeneutics.* New Haven: Yale University Press.

Grondin, Jean. 2003. *The Philosophy of Gadamer.* Oxford: Routledge Press.

Guyatt, Gordan. 2000. "Making Sense of Quality-of-Life Data." *Medical Care* 38 (9): II175–II179.

Guyatt, Gordan H., John Cairns, David Churchill, Deborah Cook, Brian Haynes, Jack Hirsh, Jan Irvine, et al. 1992. "Evidence-Based Medicine. A New Approach to Teaching the Practice of Medicine." *JAMA* 268 (17): 2420–25.

Guyatt, Gordan H., David H. Feeny, and Donald L. Patrick. 1993. "Measuring Health-Related Quality of Life." *Annals of Internal Medicine* 118 (8): 622–29.

Habermas, Jürgen. 1990. *Moral Consciousness and Communicative Action.* Translated by Christian Lenhardt and Shierry Weber Nicholsen. Cambridge, MA: MIT Press.

Hagquist, Curt. 2019. "Explaining Differential Item Functioning Focusing on the Crucial Role of External Information: An Example from the Measurement of Adolescent Mental Health." *BMC Medical Research* 19: 185.

Hagquist, Curt and David Andrich. 2017. "Recent Advances in Analysis of Differential Item Functioning in Health Research Using the Rasch Model." *Health and Quality of Life Outcomes* 15: 181.

Harding, Sandra. 1986. *The Science Question in Feminism.* Ithaca, NY: Cornell University Press.

Harding, Sandra. 2015. *Objectivity and Diversity: Another Logic of Scientific Research.* Chicago: University of Chicago Press.

Hausman, Daniel. 2015. *Valuing Health: Well-Being, Freedom, and Suffering.* Oxford: Oxford University Press.

Haybron, Daniel. 2008. *The Pursuit of Unhappiness: The Elusive Psychology of Well-Being.* Oxford: Oxford University Press.

Health Service Executive (HSE). 2020. "Overview Hip Replacement." Last modified December 22, 2020. https://www2.hse.ie/conditions/hip-replacement/#:~:text=Adults%20of%20any%20age%20can,ages%20of%2060%20and%2080.

Hegel, Georg Wilhelm Fredrich. 1809/1979. *Phenomenology of Sprit.* Translated by Arnold V. Miller. Oxford: Oxford University Press.

Heidegger, Martin. 1927/1996. *Being and Time.* Translated by Joan Stambaugh. Albany: SUNY Press.

Ho, Anita. 2001. "Trusting Experts and Epistemic Humility." *International Journal of Feminist Approaches to Bioethics* 4: 102–23.

Hobart, Jeremy C. and Stefan J. Cano. 2009. "Improving the Evaluation of Therapeutic Interventions in Multiple Sclerosis: The Role of New Psychometric Methods." *Health Technology Assessment* 13 (12): iii, ix–x, 1–177.

Hobart, Jeremy C., Stefan J. Cano, John P. Zajicek, and Alan J. Thompson. 2007. "Rating Scales as Outcome Measures for Clinical Trials in Neurology: Problems, Solutions and Recommendations." *Lancet Neurology* 6 (12): 1094–105.

Holman, Bennett and Justin P. Bruner. 2015. "The Problem of Intransigently Biased Agents." *Philosophy of Science* 82 (5): 956–68.

Holman, Bennett and Kevin C. Elliot. 2018. "The Promise and Perils of Industry-Funded Science." *Philosophy Compass* 13 (11): e12544.

Holman, Bennett. 2015. "The Fundamental Antagonism: Science and Commerce in Medical Epistemology." PhD diss., University of California, Irvine.

Holman, Bennett. 2019. "Philosophers on Drugs." *Synthese* 196 (11): 4363–90.

Holman, Bennett and Sally Geislar. 2018. "Sex Drugs and Corporate Ventriloquism: How to Evaluate Science Policies Intended to Manage Industry-Funded Bias." *Philosophy of Science* 85 (5): 869–81.

Howick, Jeremy, Paul Glasziou, and Jeffrey Aronson. 2010. "Evidence-Based Mechanistic Reasoning." *Journal of the Royal Society of Medicine* 103 (11): 433–41.

Hunt, Sonja M. 1997. "The Problem of Quality of Life." *Quality of Life Research* 6: 205–12.

Institute of Medicine. 2001. *Crossing the Quality Chasm: A New Health System for the 21st Century*. Washington, DC: National Academy Press.

Jaeschke, Roman, Joel Singer, and Gordan Guyatt. 1989. "Measurement of Health Status: Ascertaining the Minimal Clinically Important Difference." *Controlled Clinical Trials* 10 (4): 407–15.

Jewson, Nicolas. 1976. "The Disappearance of the Sick-Man from Medical Cosmology, 1770–1870." *Sociology* 10 (2): 225–44.

Joyce, Charles Richard Boddington, Hannah M. McGee, and Ciaran A. O'Boyle. 1999. *Quality of Life in Individual Quality of Life: Approaches to Conceptualization and Assessment*. Amsterdam: Harwood Academic Publishers.

Kant, Immanuel. 1781/1999. *The Critique of Pure Reason*. Translated and edited by Paul Guyer and Allen W. Wood. Cambridge: Cambridge University Press.

Kantrowitz, Arthur. 1967. "Proposal for an Institution for Scientific Judgment." *Science* 156 (3776): 763–64.

Keats, John A. 1967. "Test Theory." *Annual Review of Psychology* 18: 217–38.

Kennedy, Ashley Graham. 2013. "Differential Diagnosis and the Suspension of Judgement." *Journal of Medicine and Philosophy* 38 (5): 487–500.

Kidd, Ian James and Havi Carel. 2017. "Epistemic Injustice and Illness." *Journal of Applied Philosophy* 34 (2): 172–90.

Kidd, Ian James and Havi Carel. 2018. "Healthcare Practice, Epistemic Injustice, and Naturalism." *Royal Institute of Philosophy Supplement* 84: 211–33.

Kitcher, Philip and Wesley Salmon. 1987. "Van Frassen on Explanation." *Journal of Philosophy* 84 (6): 315–30.

Krantz, David H., R. Duncan Luce, Patrick Suppes, and Amos Tversky. 1971. *Foundations of Measurement*. Vol. 1: *Additive and Polynomial Representations*. New York: Academic Press.

Kuhn, Thomas. 1977. "Second Thoughts on Paradigms." In Kuhn, *The Essential Tension: Selected Studies in Scientific Tradition and Change*, 293–319. Chicago: Chicago University Press.

Kyngdon, Andrew. 2008a. "Conjoint Measurement, Error and the Rasch Model: A Reply to Michell, and Borsboom and Zand Scholten." *Theory & Psychology* 18 (1): 125–31.

Kyngdon, Andrew. 2008b. "The Rasch Model from the Perspective of the Representational Theory of Measurement." *Theory & Psychology* 18 (1): 89–109.

Lammi, Walter. 1991. "Hans-Georg Gadamer's 'Correction' of Heidegger." *Journal of the History of Ideas* 52 (3): 487–507.

Leplège, Alain and Sonia Hunt. 1997. "The Problem of Quality of Life in Medicine." *Journal of the American Medical Association* 278 (1): 47–50.

Lloyd, Elisabeth. 1995. "Objectivity and the Double Standard of Feminist Epistemologies." *Synthese* 104 (3): 351–81.

Lokhorst, Max M., Sophie E. R. Horbach, Danny Young-Afat, Merel L. E. Stor, Lotte Haverman, Phyllis Spuls, Chantal M. A. M. van der Horst, and the Outcomes Measures for Vascular Malformations (OVAMA) Steering Group. 2021. "Development of a Condition-Specific Patient-Reported Outcome Measure for Measuring Symptoms and Appearance in Vascular Malformations: The OVAMA Questionnaire." *British Journal of Dermatology* 185 (4): 797–803.

Longino, Helen E. 1990. *Science as Social Knowledge*. Princeton: Princeton University Press.

Longino, Helen E. 2002. *The Fate of Knowledge*. Princeton: Princeton University Press.

Lord, Frederic M. and Melvin Robert Novick. 2008. *Statistical Theories of Mental Test Scores*. Charlotte, NC: Information Age Publishing.

Lorde, Audrey. 1984. *Sister Outsider: Essays and Speeches*. Berkeley: Crossing Press.

Loscalzo, Matthew J. 2008. "Palliative Care: An Historical Perspective." *Hematology, American Society of Hematology Education Program* 1: 465.

Luce, Bryan R., Joan M. Weschler and Carol Underwood. 1989. "The Use of Quality-of-Life Measures in the Private Sector." In *Quality of Life and Technology Assessment: Monograph of the Council on Health Care Technology*, edited by Frederick Mosteller and Jennifer Falotico-Taylor, 55–64. Washington, DC: National Academies Press.

Luce, R. Duncan and John W. Tukey. 1964. "Simultaneous Conjoint Measurement: A New Type of Fundamental Measurement." *Journal of Mathematical Psychology* 1: 1–27.

Lupton, Deborah. 2014. "The Commodification of Patient Opinion: The Digital Patient Experience Economy in the Age of Big Data." *Sociology of Health & Illness* 36 (6): 856–69.

Lynch, Grey. 2021. "Gadamer's Aspectival Realism." *Ergo* 7.

MacIntyre, Alasdair. 1981. "The Nature of the Virtues." *Hastings Center Report* 11 (2): 27–34.

Mallinson, Sara. 2002. "Listening to Respondents: Assessment of the Short-Form 36 Health Status Questionnaire." *Social Science & Medicine* 54 (1): 11–21.

Mayo, Nancy. 2015. *ISOQOL Dictionary of Quality of Life and Health Outcomes Measurement*. Milwaukee: ISOQOL.

Mazor, Joseph. 2013. "The Child's Interest and the Case for the Permissibility of Male Infant Circumcision." *Journal of Medical Ethics* 39 (7): 421–28.

McClimans, Leah. 2010a. "Towards Self-Determination in Quality of Life Research." *Medicine, Health Care and Philosophy* 13: 67–76.

McClimans, Leah. 2010b. "A Theoretical Framework for Patient-Reported Outcome Measures." *Theoretical Medicine and Bioethics* 31 (3): 225–40.

McClimans, Leah. 2011. "The Art of Asking Questions." *International Journal of Philosophical Studies* 19 (4): 521–38.

McClimans, Leah. 2011. "Interpretability, Validity and the Minimum Important Difference." *Theoretical Medicine and Bioethics* 32: 389–401.

McClimans, Leah. 2016. "A Dialogic Approach to Narrative Medicine." In *Inheriting Gadamer: New Directions in Philosophical Hermeneutics*, edited by Georgia Warnke, 203–17. Edinburgh: University of Edinburgh Press.

McClimans, L. 2017. Health Measurement, Industry and Science. In *Philosophical Issues in Pharmaceutics: Use, Dispensing and Development*, edited by Dien Ho, pp. 93–108. Springer.

McClimans, Leah, Jerome Bickenbach, Marjan Westerman, Licia Carlson, David Wasserman, and Carolyn E. Schwartz. 2012. "Philosophical Perspectives on Response Shift." *Quality of Life Research* 22: 1871–78.

McClimans, Leah and John Browne. 2011. "Choosing a Patient-Reported Outcome Measure." *Theoretical Medicine and Bioethics* 32: 47–60.

McClimans, Leah and John Browne. 2012. "Quality of Life Is a Process Not an Outcome." *Theoretical Medicine and Bioethics* 33 (4): 279–92.

McClimans, Leah, John Browne, and Stefan Cano. 2017. "Clinical Outcome Measurement: Models, Theory, Psychometrics and Practice." *Studies in the History and Philosophy of Science* 65: 67–73.

McHorney, Colleen A. and Alvin R. Tarlov. 1995. "Individual-Patient Monitoring in Clinical Practice: Are Available Health Status Surveys Adequate?" *Quality of Life Research* 4: 293–307.

McKenna, Stephen. 2011. "Measurement Patient-Reported Outcomes: Moving beyond Misplaced Sense to Hard Science." *BMC Medicine* 9: 86.

Mellenbergh, Gideon. 1989. "Item Bias and Item Response Theory." *International Journal of Educational Research* 13 (2): 127–43.

Messick, Samuel. 1980. "Test Validity and the Ethics of Assessment." *American Psychologist* 35 (11): 1012–27.

Michell, Joel. 2000. "Normal Science, Pathological Science and Psychometrics." *Theory & Psychology* 10: 639–67.

Michell, Joel. 2008. "Conjoint Measurement and the Rasch Paradox: A Response to Kyngdon." *Theory & Psychology* 18 (1): 119–24.

Mills, Charles. 1997. *The Racial Contract*. Ithaca, NY: Cornell University Press.

Mokkink, Lidwine B., Caroline B. Terwee, Donald L. Patrick, Jordi Alonso, Paul W. Statford, Dirk L. Knol, Lex M. Bouter, and Henrica C. W. de Vet. 2010. "The COSMIN Checklist for Assessing the Methodological Quality of Studies on Measurement Properties of Health Status Measurement Instruments: An International Delphi Study." *Quality of life Research* 19 (4): 539–49.

Mokkink, Lidwine, Cecilia A. C. Prinsen, Donald L. Patrick, Jordi Alonso, Lex M. Bouter, Henrica C.W. de Vet, and Caroline B Terwee. 2019. "COSMIN Study Design checklist for Patient-Reported Outcomes Measurement Instruments." https://www.cosmin.nl/tools/checklists-assessing-methodological-study-qualities/.

Mol, Annemarie. 2008. *The Logic of Care: Health and the Problem of Patient Choice*. New York: Routledge.

Monk, Kendra. 2014. "Making the Cut: A Phenomenological Study of the Parental Decision-Making Process for Neonatal Circumcision." Master's thesis, University of Manitoba.

Monticone, Marco, Giorgio Ferriero, Andrea Giordano, Calogero Foti, and Franco Franchignoni. 2020. "Rasch Analysis of the Incontinence Impact Questionnaire Short Version (IIQ-7) in Women with Urinary Incontinence." *International Journal of Rehabilitation Research* 43 (3): 261–65.

Mota, Rubén Ernesto Mújica. 2013. "Cost Effectiveness Analysis of Early versus Late Total Hip Replacement in Italy." *Value in Health* 16 (2): 267–79.

Mukherjee, Siddhartha. 2010. *The Emperor of All Maladies*. New York: Scribner.

Nagel, Thomas. 1973. "Rawls on Justice." *Philosophical Review* 82 (2): 220–34.

Navarra, Sandra V., Robelle M. D. V. Tanangunan, Rachel A. Mikolaitis-Preuss, Mark Kosinski, Joel A. Block, and Meenakshi Jolly. 2013. "Cross-Cultural Validation of a

Disease-Specific Patient-Reported Outcomes Measure for Lupus in the Philippines." *Lupus* 22 (3): 262–67.

Ng, Weiting, William Tov, Ruut Veenhoven, Sebastiaan Rothmann, Maria José Chambel, Sufen Chen, Matthew L. Cole, et al. 2021. "In Memory of Edward Diener: Reflections on His Career, Contributions, and the Sciences of Happiness." *Frontiers in Psychology* 12: 706447.

NHS. "Patient Reported Outcome Measures (PROMS)." Accessed June 17, 2023. https://www.england.nhs.uk/statistics/statistical-work-areas/proms/.

Nunnery, Jum C and Ira H. Bernstein. 1994. *Psychometric Theory*. 3rd ed. New York: McGraw-Hill.

Nussbaum, Martha. 2000. *Women and Human Development: The Capabilities Approach.* Cambridge: Cambridge University Press.

O'Boyle, Ciaran, Hannah McGee, Anne Hickey, C. R. B. Joyce, John Browne, Kevin O'Malley, and Beat Hiltbrunner. 1993. *The Schedule for the Evaluation of Individual Quality of Life (SEIQoL). Administrative Manual*. Dublin: Royal College of Surgeons in Ireland.

Olsen, Jørn and IEA European Questionnaire Group. 1998. "Epidemiology Deserves Better Questionnaires." *International Journal of Epidemiology* 27 (6): 935.

Oort, Frans. 2005. "Using Structural Equation Modeling to Detect Response Shifts and True Change." *Quality of Life Research* 14 (3): 587–98.

Oort, Frans, Mechteld Visser, and Mirjam Sprangers. 2009. "Formal Definitions of Measurement Bias and Explanation Bias Clarify Measurement and Conceptual Perspectives on Response Shift." *Journal of Clinical Epidemiology* 62 (11): 1126–37.

Oreskes, Naomi and Erik M. Conway. 2010. *Merchants of Doubt: How a Handful of Scientists Obscured the Truth on Issues from Tobacco Smoke to Climate Change*. London: Bloomsbury Publishing.

Organization for Economic Cooperation and Development. 2017. Ministerial Statement "The Next Generation of Health Reforms." Accessed June 20, 2023. https://www.oecd.org/newsroom/oecd-health-ministerial-statement-the-next-generation-of-health-reforms.htm.

Oswald, Andrew J. 2008. "On the Curvature of the Reporting Function from Objective Reality to Subjective Feelings." *Economic Letters* 110: 369–72.

Patel, Kavita K., David L. Veestra, and Donald L. Patrick. 2003. "A Review of Selected Patient-Generated Outcome Measures and Their Application in Clinical Trials." *Value in Health* 6 (5): 595–603.

Paul, Laurie A. 2014. *Transformative Experience*. Oxford: Oxford University Press.

Perline, Richard, Benjamin D. Wright, and Howard Wainer. 1979. "The Rasch Model as Additive Conjoint Measurement." *Applied Psychological Measurement* 3: 237–55.

Petrillo, Jennifer, Stefan J. Cano, Lori D. McLeod, and Cheryl D. Coon. 2014. "Using Classical Test Theory, Item Response Theory and Rasch Measurement Theory to Evaluate Patient-Reported Outcomes Measures: A Comparison of Worked Examples." *Value in Health* 18 (1): 25–34.

Pols, Jeannette. 2006. "Accounting and Washing: Good Care in Long-Term Psychiatry." *Science, Technology, & Human Values* 31 (4): 409–30.

Porter, Theodore M. 1985. "The Mathematics of Society: Variation and Error in Quetelet's Statistics." *British Journal for the History of Science* 18 (1): 51–69.

Porter, Theodore M. 1995. *Trust in Numbers*. Princeton: Princeton University Press.

Pusic, Andrea L., Anne F. Klassen, Amie M. Scott, Jennifer A. Klok, Peter G. Cordeiro, and Stefan J. Cano. 2009. "Development of a New Patient-Reported Outcome Measure for Breast Surgery: The BREAST-Q." *Plastic Reconstructive Surgery* 124 (2): pp 345–53.

Putnick, Diane, L., and Marc H. Bornstein. 2016. "Measurement Invariance Conventions and Reporting: The State of the Art and Future Directions for Psychological Research." *Developmental Review* 41: 71–90.

Rapkin, Bruce D., Iliana Garcia, Wesley Michael, Jie Zhang, and Carolyn E. Schwartz. 2017. "Distinguishing Appraisal and Personality Influences on Quality of Life in Chronic Illness: Introducing the Quality-of-Life Appraisal Profile Version 2." *Quality of Life Research* 26 (10): 2815–29.

Rapkin, Bruce D., Iliana Garcia, Wesley Michael, Jie Zhang, and Carolyn E. Schwartz. 2018. "Development of a Practical Outcome Measure to Account for Individual Differences in Quality-of-Life Appraisal: The Brief Appraisal Inventory." *Quality of Life Research* 27 (3): 823–33.

Rapkin, Bruce D. and Carolyn E. Schwartz. 2004. "Toward a Theoretical Model of Quality-of-Life Appraisal: Implications of Findings from Studies of Response Shift." *Health and Quality of Life Outcomes* 2: 14.

Rapkin, Bruce D. and Carolyn E. Schwartz. 2019. "Advancing Quality-of-Life Research by Deepening Our Understanding of Response Shift: A Unifying Theory of Appraisal." *Quality of Life Research* 28 (11): 2623–30.

Rapkin, Bruce D. and Carolyn E. Schwartz. 2021. "What Should Progress in Response-Shift Research Look Like?" *Quality of Life Research* 30 (12): 3359–61.

Rasch, Georg. 1960. *Probabilistic Models for Some Intelligence and Attainment Tests.* Copenhagen: Danish Institute for Education Research.

Rawls, John. 1999. *A Theory of Justice.* Rev ed. Cambridge, MA: Belknap Press of Harvard University Press.

Reiss, Julian. 2020. "What Are the Drivers of Induction? Towards a Material Theory+." *Studies in History and Philosophy of Science Part A* 83 (October): 8–16.

Robeyns, Ingrid, and Morten Fibieger Byskov. 2020. "The Capability Approach." In *The Stanford Encyclopedia of Philosophy* (Winter 2021 ed.), edited by Edward N. Zalta and Uri Nodelman. https://plato.stanford.edu/archives/sum2023/entries/capability-approach/.

Rorty, Richard. 2004. "Being That Can Be Understood Is Language." In *Gadamer's Repercussions: Reconsidering Philosophical Hermeneutics*, edited by Bruce Krajewski, 21–30. Berkeley: University of California Press.

Rothman, David. 1992. *Strangers at the Bedside A History of How Law and Bioethics Transformed Medical Decision Making.* New York: Basic Books.

Rothman, Margaret, Laurie Burke, Pennifer Erickson, Nancy Klein Leidy, Donald L. Patrick, and Charles D. Petrie. 2009. "Use of Existing Patient-Reported Outcome (PRO) Instruments and Their Modification: The ISPOR Good Research Practices for Evaluating and Documenting Content Validity for the Use of Existing Instruments and Their Modification PRO Task Force Report." *Value in Health* 12 (8): 1075–83.

Rothrock, Nan E., Karen Kaiser, and David Cella. 2011. "Developing a Valid Patient-Reported Outcome Measure." *Clinical Pharmacology & Therapeutics* 90 (5): 737–42.

Rusch, Thomas, Paul Benjamin Lowry, Patrick Mair, and Horst Treiblmaier. 2017. "Breaking Free from the Limitations of Classical Test Theory: Developing and Measuring Information Systems Scales Using Item Response Theory." *Information & Management* 54 (2): 189–203.

Ruta, Danny A, Andrew M. Garratt, Mhoira Leng, Ian T. Russell, and Lesley M. MacDonald. 1994. "A New Approach to the Measurement of Quality of Life: The Patient-Generated Index." *Medical Care* 32 (11): 1109–26.

Sajobi, Tolulope T., Ronak Brahambatt, Lisa M. Lix, Bruno D. Zumbo, and Richard Sawatzky. 2018. "Scoping Review of Response Shift Methods: Current Reporting Practices and Recommendations." *Quality of Life Research* 27 (4): 1133–46.

Scanlon, Thomas M. 1998. *What We Owe Each Other*. Cambridge, MA: Belknap Press of Harvard University Press.

Schimmack, Ulrich. 2021. "The Validation Crisis in Psychology." *Meta-Psychology* 5.

Schwartz, Adina. 1973. "Moral Neutrality and Primary Goods." *Ethics* 83 (4): 294–307.

Schwartz, Carolyn E., Elena M. Andresen, Margaret Nosek, and Gloria Krahn. 2007. "Response Shift Theory: Important Implications for Measuring Quality of Life in People with Disability." *Archives of Physical Medicine and Rehabilitation* 88 (4): 529–36.

Schwartz, Carolyn E. and Bruce Rapkin D. 2004. "Reconsidering the Psychometrics of Quality of Life Assessment in Light of Response Shift and Appraisal." *Health and Quality of Life Outcomes* 2 (1): 16.

Schwartz, Carolyn E., and Mirjam A. G. Sprangers. 1999. "Methodological Approaches for Assessing Response Shift in Longitudinal Health-Related Quality-of-Life Research." *Social Science & Medicine* 48 (11): 1531–48.

Schwartz, Carolyn E., Roland Stark, and Bruce D. Rapkin. 2020. "Capturing Patient Experience: Does Quality of Life Appraisal Entail a New Class of Measurement?" *Journal of Patient-Reported Outcomes* 4: 85.

Schwartz, Carolyn E., Roland Stark, and Bruce D. Rapkin. 2021. "Creating Idiometric Short-Form Measures of Cognitive Appraisal: Balancing Theory and Pragmatics." *Journal of Patient-Recorded Outcomes* 5: 57.

Schwartz, Carolyn E., Brian Stucky, Wesley Michael, and Bruce D. Rapkin. 2020. "Does Response Shift Impact Interpretation of Change Even among Scales Developed Using Item Response Theory?" *Journal of Patient Reported Outcomes* 4 (1): 8.

Sébille, Véronique, Lisa M. Lix, Olawale F. Ayilara, Tolulope T. Sajobi, A. Cecile J. W. Janssens, Richard Sawatzky, Mirjam A. G. Sprangers, Mathilde G. E. Verdam, and the Response Shift–in Sync Working Group. 2021. "Critical Examination of Current Response Shift Methods and Proposal for Advancing New Methods." *Quality of Life Research* 30 (12): 3325–42.

Sen, A. 1979. *"Equality of What?" The Tanner Lecture on Human Values*. Stanford: Stanford University.

Sen, Amartya. 1984. "Well-Being, Agency and Freedom: The Dewey Lectures 1984." *Journal of Philosophy* 82 (4): 169–221.

Sen, Amartya. 1993. "Capability and Well-Being." In *The Quality of Life*, edited by Martha Nussbaum and Amartya Sen, 30–53. Oxford: Clarendon Press.

Sismondo, Sergio. 2007. "Ghost Management: How Much of the Medical Literature Is Shaped behind the Scenes by the Pharmaceutical Industry?" *PloS Medicine* 4 (9): e286.

Sismondo, Sergio. 2018. *Ghost-Managed Medicine: Big Pharm's Invisible Hands*. Manchester: Mattering Press.

Sismondo, Sergio and Mathieu Doucet. 2010. "Publication Ethics and the Ghost Management of Medical Publication." *Bioethics* 24 (6): 273–83.

Sismondo, Sergio and Scott Howard Nicholson. 2009. "Publication Planning 101." *Journal of Pharmacy and Pharmaceutical Sciences* 12 (3): 273–79.

Skorupska, Katarzyna, Magdalena Emilia Grybowska, Agnieszka Kubik-Komar, Tomasz Rechberger, and Pawel Miotla. 2021. "Identification of the Urogenital Distress Inventory-6 and the Incontinence Impact Questionnaire-7 Cutoff Scores in Urinary Incontinent Women." *Health and Quality of Life Outcomes* 19: 87.

Snow, Rosamund, Charlotte Humphrey, and Jane Sandall. 2013. "What Happens When Patients Know More Than Their Doctors? Experience of Health Interactions after Diabetes Patient Education: A Qualitative Patient-Led Study." *BMJ Open* 3 (11): e003583.

Sontag, Susan. 1978. *Illness as Metaphor*. New York: Farrar, Straus, and Giroux.

Spitzer, W. O., A. J. Dobson, J. Hall, E. Chesterman, J. Levi, R. Shepherd, R. N. Battista, and B. R. Catchlove. 1981. *Quality of Life Index (QL-Index)* [database record]. APA PsycTests.

Sprangers, Mirjam, Tolulope Sajobi, Antoine Vanier, Nancy Mayo, Richard Sawatzky, Lisa Lix, Frans Oort, and Véronique Sébille. 2021. "Response Shift in Results of Patient-Reported Outcome Measures: A Commentary to The Response Shift–in Sync Working Group Initiative." *Quality of Life Research* 30 (12): 3299–308.

Sprangers, Mirjam and Carolyn E. Schwartz. 1999. "Integrating Response Shift into Health-Related Quality-of-Life Research: A Theoretical Model." *Social Science & Medicine* 48 (11): 1507–15.

Stenner, A. Jackson, William P. Fisher Jr., Mark H. Stone, and Donald Burdick. 2013. "Causal Rasch Models." *Frontiers in Psychology* 4: 536.

Stirling, Jeannette. 2010. *Representing Epilepsy: Myth and Matter*. Liverpool: Liverpool University Press.

Streiner, David L. and Geoffrey R. Norman. 2003. *Health Measurement Scales: A Practical Guide to Their Development and Use*. 3rd ed. Oxford: Oxford University Press.

Sullivan, Shannon and Nancy Tuana, eds. 2007. *Race and Epistemologies of Ignorance*. New York: SUNY Press.

Svoboda, Steven J., Peter W. Adler, and Robert S. Van Howe. 2016. "Circumcision Is Unethical and Unlawful." *Journal of Law, Medicine and Ethics* 44 (2): 263–82.

Swartz, Richard J., Caroline E. Schwartz, Ethan Basch, Li Cai, Diane L. Fairclough, Lori McLeod, Tito R. Mendoza, Bruce D. Rapkin, and SAMSI Psychometric Program Longitudinal Assessment of Patient-Reported Outcomes Working Group. 2011. "The King's Foot of Patient-Reported Outcomes: Current Practices and New Developments for the Measurement of Change." *Quality of Life Research* 20: 1159–67.

Tal, Eran. "Measurement in Science." In *The Stanford Encyclopedia of Philosophy* (Fall 2020 ed.), edited by Edward N. Zalta. https://plato.stanford.edu/archives/fall2020/entries/measurement-science/.

Tal, Eran. 2011. "How Accurate Is the Standard Second?" *Philosophy of Science* 78 (5): 1082–96.

Tal, Eran. 2016. "Making Time: A Study in the Epistemology of Measurement." *British Journal for the Philosophy of Science* 67 (1): 297–335.

Tal, Eran. 2017. "Calibration: Modeling the Measurement Process." *Studies in History and Philosophy of Science Part A* 65–66: 33–45.

Tang, Jessica A., Oh Taemin, Justin K. Scheer, and Andrew T. Parsa. 2014. "The Current Trend of Administering a Patient-Generated Oncological Setting: A Systematic Review." *Oncology Reviews* 8: 245.

Taylor, Charles. 1985. "Self-Interpreting Animals." In Taylor, *Human Agency and Language, Philosophical Papers*, vol. 1, 45–76. Cambridge: Cambridge University Press.

Terwee, Caroline, Sandra D. M. Bot, Michael R. de Boer, Daniëlle A. W. M. van der Windt, Dirk L. Knoll, Joost Dekker, Lex M. Bouter, and Henrica C. W. de Vet. 2007. "Quality Criteria Were Proposed for Measurement Properties of Health Status Questionnaires." *Journal of Clinical Epidemiology* 60 (1): 34–42.

The Lancet. 2018. "Normalising Menstruation, Empowering Girls." *Lancet Child & Adolescent Health* 2 (6): 379.

Thomas, Rachel. "Why Women Get Overlooked in Healthcare." *Tilted: A Lean In Podcast.* December 11, 2008. https://www.stitcher.com/podcast/lean-in/tilted-a-lean-in-podc ast/e/57663934.

Thompson, Jake W. 2018. "Construct Irrelevance." In *The Sage Encyclopedia of Educational Research, Measurement, and Evaluation,* edited by Bruce B. Frey. Sage Publications. https://sk.sagepub.com/reference/sage-encyclopedia-of-educational-research-meas urement-evaluation/i5811.xml.

Timmerman, Carsten. 2013. "'Just Give Me the Best Quality of Life Questionnaire': The Karnofsky Scale and the History of Quality of Life Measurements in Cancer Trials." *Chronic Illness* 9 (3): 179–90.

Timmermans, Stefan and Marc Berg. 2003. *The Gold Standard: The Challenge of Evidence-Based Medicine and Standardization in Health Care.* Philadelphia: Temple University Press.

Traub, Ross E. 1997. "Classical Test Theory in Historical Perspective." *Educational Measurement: Issues and Practice* 16 (4): 8–14.

Trujols, Joan and Maria J. Portella. 2013. "Not All PROMs Reflect Patients' Perspectives." *British Medical Journal* 346: f1552.

Paine, Mark Bigelow. 1912. *Mark Twain A Biography: The Personal and Literary Life of Samuel Langhorne Clemens,* Vol. III. New York: Harper and Brothers, 1341.

Uebersax, John S., Jean F. Wyman, Sally A. Shucker, Donna K. McClish, and Andrew Fantl. 1995. "Short Forms to Assess Life Quality and Symptom Distress for Urinary Incontinence in Women: The Incontinence Impact Questionnaire and the Urogenital Distress Inventory. Continence Program for Women Research Group." *Neurourology and Urodynamics* 14 (2): 131–9.

United Nations. 2022. "Removing the Shame and Stigma from Menstruation." Last modified July 8, 2022. https://www.ohchr.org/en/stories/2022/07/removing-shame-and-sti gma-menstruation.

United Nations Women. 2019. "Infographic: End the Stigma. Period." Last modified October 6, 2019. https://www.unwomen.org/en/digital-library/multimedia/2019/10/ infographic-periods.

Vaccarella, Maria. 2011. "Narrative Epileptology." *The Lancet* 377: 460–61.

van Fraassen, Bas. 1980. *The Scientific Image.* New York: Oxford University Press.

van Fraassen, Bas. 2008. *Scientific Representations: Paradoxes of Perspective.* Oxford: Oxford University Press.

van Loon, Miriam, Karen M. van Leeuwen, Raymond W. Ostelo, Judith E. Bosmans, and Guy Antonie Marie Widdershoven. 2018. "Quality of Life in a Broader Perspective: Does ASCOT Reflect the Capability Approach?" *Quality of Life Research* 27 (5): 1181–89.

VandenBos, Gary R., ed. 2015. *APA Dictionary of Psychology.* 2nd ed. Washington, DC: American Psychological Association.

Vanier, Antoine, Bruno Falissard, Véronique Sébille, and Jean-Benoit Hardouin. 2018. "The Complexity of Interpreting Changes Observed over Time in Health-Related Quality of Life: A Short Overview of 15 Years of Research on Response Shift Theory." In

Perceived Health and Adaptation in Chronic Disease, edited by Francis Guillemin, Alain Leplège, Serge Briancon, Elisabeth Spitz, and Joel Coste, 202–30. New York: Routledge.

Vanier, Antoine, Frans Oort, Leah McClimans, Nikki Ow, Bernice Gulek, Jan Böhnke, Mirjam Sprangers, Véronique Sébille, and Nancy Mayo. 2021. "Response Shift in Patient-Reported Outcomes: Definition, Theory, and a Revised Model." *Quality of Life Research* 30 (12): 1–14.

Vaughan, Louella and John Browne. 2022. "Reconfiguring Emergency and Acute Services: Time to Pause and Reflect." *British Medical Journal Quality & Safety* 32: 185–88.

Verkerk, Mirian, J. J. van Busschbach, and E. D. Karssing. 2001. "Health-Related Quality of Life Research and the Capability Approach of Amartya Sen." *Quality of Life Research* 10 (1): 49–55.

Visser, Mechteld, Frans Oort, and Mirjam Sprangers. 2005. "Methods to Detect Response Shift in Quality of Life Data: A Convergent Validity Study." *Quality of Life Research* 14 (3): 629–39.

Wachterhauser, Brice. 1994. "Gadamer's Realism: The 'Belongingness' of World and Reality." In *Hermeneutics and Truth: Studies in Phenomenal and Existential Philosophy*, edited by Brice Wachterhauser, 148–71. Evanston, IL: Northwestern University Press.

Wachterhauser, Brice. 1999. *Beyond Being: Gadamer's Post-Platonic Hermeneutic Ontology*. Evanston, IL: Northwestern University Press.

Wachterhauser, Brice. 2002. "Getting It Right: Relativism, Realism and Truth." In *The Cambridge Companion to Gadamer* edited by Robert J. Dostal, 52–78. New York: Cambridge University Press.

Ware, John E. and Cathy Donald Sherbourne. 1992. "The MOS 36-Item Short-Form Health Survey (SF-36): I. Conceptual Framework and Item Selection." *Medical Care* 30 (6): 473–83.

Warnke, Georgia. 1999. *Gadamer: Hermeneutics, Tradition and Reason*. Oxford: Polity Press.

Warnke, Georgia. 2011. "The Hermeneutic Circle versus Dialogue." *Review of Metaphysics* 65 (1): 91–112.

Warnke, Georgia. 2014. "Hermeneutics and Feminism." In *The Routledge Companion to Hermeneutics*, edited by Jeff Malpas and Hans-Helmuth Gander, 644–59. New York: Routledge.

Watt, Torquil, Jakob Bue Bjorner, Mogens Groenvold, Åse Krogh Rasmussen, Steen Joop Bonnema, Laszlo Hegedüs, and Ulla Feldt-Rasmussen. 2009. "Establishing Construct Validity for the Thyroid-Specific Patient Reported Outcome Measure (ThyPro): An Initial Examination." *Quality of Life Research* 18 (4): 483–96.

Wellmer, Albrecht. 1974. *Critical Theory of Society*. Translated by John Cumming. New York: Seabury Press.

Westerman, Marjan, Tony Hak, Mirjam Sprangers, Harry Groen, Garrit van der Wal, and Anne-Mei The. 2008. "Listen to Their Answers! Response Behaviour in the Measurement of Physical and Role Functioning." *Quality of Life Research* 17 (4): 549–58.

Wiering, Bianca, Dolf de Boer, and Diana Delnoij. 2017. "Patient Involvement in the Development of Patient-Reported Outcome Measures: The Developers' Perspective." *BMC Health Services Research* 17: 635.

Wilde, Meriel and Cheryl Haslam. 1996. "Living with Epilepsy: A Qualitative Study Investigating the Experience of Young People Attending Outpatients Clinics in Leicester." *Seizure* 5 (1): 63–72.

Wilson, Mark. 2005. *Constructing Measures: An Item Response Modeling Approach.* Mahwah, NJ: Lawrence Erlbaum Associates.

Wilson, Mark. 2013. "Using the Concept of a Measurement System to Characterize Measurement Models Used in Psychometrics." *Measurement* 46 (9): 3766–74.

World Health Organization. 2022. *International Classification of Diseases and Related Health Problems.* 11th ed. https://icd.who.int/browse11/l-m/en.

Wu, Albert W., Claire Snyder, Carolyn M. Clancy, and Donald M. Steinwachs. 2010. "Adding the Patient Perspective to Comparative Effectiveness Research." *Health Affairs* 29 (10): 1863–71.

Index

For the benefit of digital users, indexed terms that span two pages (e.g., 52–53) may, on occasion, appear on only one of those pages.